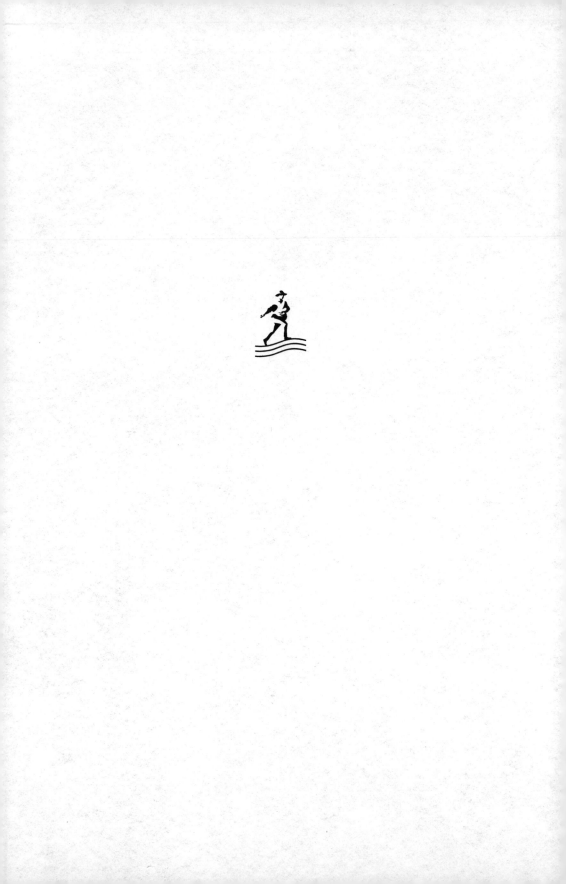

Also by Edward Humes

Mean Justice

No Matter How Loud I Shout

Mississippi Mud

Murderer With a Badge

Buried Secrets

Baby ER

The Heroic Doctors and Nurses Who
Perform Medicine's Tiniest Miracles

Edward Humes

Simon & Schuster

NEW YORK • TORONTO • LONDON • SYDNEY • SINGAPORE

SIMON & SCHUSTER
Rockefeller Center
1230 Avenue of the Americas
New York, New York 10020

Designed by Lisa Chovnick

Manufactured in the United States of America

1   3   5   7   9   10   8   6   4   2

Library of Congress Cataloging-in-Publication Data
Humes, Edward.
Baby ER : the heroic doctors and nurses who perform medicine's tiniest miracles / Edward Humes.
p. cm.
1. Neonatal intensive care—Popular works. 2. Neonatal emergencies—Popular works.
I. Title: Baby ER. II. Title.

RJ253.5 .H86 2000
618.92'01—dc21   00-061870

ISBN 0-684-86410-X

To Gabrielle and Eben

Baby ER

Preface

THIS BOOK OWES ITS ORIGINS TO THE WORST WEEK MY FAMILY HAS ever experienced—the seven terrible days in 1992 our newborn daughter, Gabrielle, spent in neonatal intensive care.

Gaby had been home barely a day when she started running a temperature and refusing to eat. To our surprise, the pediatrician did not dispense Tylenol and the usual advice when we brought her in; he sent us to the hospital for an emergency admission. "A fever in a newborn is not like a fever in an older child," Dr. John Samson told us. "She needs to go to the hospital. Right now. I'll call ahead to arrange it and meet you there."

Dr. Samson does not mince words. He has been a pediatrician for a quarter of a century, and he has thirteen children of his own, which is to say he has seen and heard it all. He took one look at Donna's and my stunned expressions, and before we could say a thing, he added with deliberate abruptness, "This is the point where most parents start to cry. And that's when I tell them, your child needs to go to the hospital now. Or she could die."

Like most new parents whose newborn children are sick, we were utterly unprepared for this verbal slap in the face. The most amazing, wonderful, miraculous day we had ever experienced was followed, a mere forty-eight hours later, by the most terrifying day of our lives.

Much of what followed is a blur to me now, but somehow we got Gaby back into her car seat and drove to the Long Beach Memorial Medical Center, rode the elevators to the second floor of the adjacent Miller Children's Hospital, and followed the signs to the Neonatal Intensive Care Unit. A nurse took her from us and walked into what appeared to be an emergency room reserved for babies, crammed with electronics and full of doctors and nurses in surgical scrubs, all of them looking intently into aquarium-sized incubators that contained some very tiny, very sick looking infants. We watched helplessly as a bewildering array of activities coalesced around our daughter, some of them recognizable—the typical weighing, measuring, blood sampling and X-raying—and some of them not.

Without fully realizing it, we had entered medicine's most cutting edge, a world we had never experienced or imagined, the most amazing part of the hospital you'll never hope to visit: the NICU. We would live there for the next week as we stood vigil, obsessively reading Gaby's chart, asking the nurses and neonatologists endless questions and watching everything, no matter how hard, even the spinal tap they gave our daughter to test for encephalitis.

We soon learned Gaby had a serious kidney infection, but it was caught in time. She responded to a course of powerful antibiotics and then, much to our relief, began eating. In retrospect, once the fear of losing our child receded and Gaby grew stronger, we realized we were among the most fortunate parents in the NICU. Most of the babies around us were tiny preemies, two- and three-pound infants dwarfed by our eight-pound daughter, whom the nurses nicknamed "Big Girl." Gaby never needed oxygen, never had to be resuscitated, had no birth defects or heart trouble or lung damage or drug addictions—none of the daunting problems afflicting most of the other babies, who were in for months, even years of recovery. Even so, I doubt that we will ever live through a harder, longer time than that awful, hot September.

It never occurred to me to write about this experience. It was too personal, too traumatic. But years later, while giving a talk about a book I had written on the children of juvenile court, I was asked what could be done to make that ailing part of the justice system work better. My answer was that the juvenile court moved too slowly, taking months to intervene in the lives of young people in crisis, when hours were called for. The juvenile court needs to work more like an emergency room, I said, acting quickly to save our troubled children before they are lost to us for good. As I uttered these words, I realized I knew a place that *did* work like that, an emergency room that moved swiftly to save our children, a fascinating, dramatic place that is in every way the antithesis of the bedraggled and defeated system of juvenile justice I had been immersed in: the NICU that had saved our daughter.

Six years after Gaby's stay there, I returned to the Neonatal Intensive Care Unit at Miller Children's Hospital, this time as a journalist and observer, where the staff, patients and many families shared with me their insights and experiences. The NICU doctors, nurses and other staff members opened their doors for me without conditions or limits, offering an unvarnished look at what they can and can't do. The parents I spent time with shared their incredible moments with me—both good and bad—with measures of candor and courage I will never forget. For this opportunity to tell their stories, I thank them all.

The events and people described in this book—the medical conditions, the patients, their families and the medical personnel—are all real and reported as faithfully as possible. Staff members and families who are named gave the author permission to do so. For reasons of privacy and in accordance with the agreement with Miller Children's Hospital granting the author access to the NICU, the names of six patients and their families have been changed. The following children's names are pseudonyms: David Rios, Baby Girl Berger, Sammy Bernard, Jessica Jones, Baby Melissa and Angela McGee.

I wish to thank the following people specifically for welcoming me into their world and thereby making this book possible: Dr. Arthur Strauss, Dr. Lupe Padilla, Dr. Jose Perez, Dr. Penny Jacinto, Dr. Steve Cho and Dr. Leonel Guajardo, the six neonatologists of the Long Beach NICU; Purificacion Tumbaga, neonatal fellow (now an attending neonatologist in Pasadena); Valerie Josephson, pediatric resident; neonatal nurses Patty Rulon, Kim Holloway, Denise Callahan, Julie France, Kim Neugebauer, Karin Nakamura, Jody King, Margie Perez, Ramona Ackerman, Kathy Hauck, Donna Prochnow, Martha Rivera, Nancy Burkey, Kathy Chao, Chris Merlo, Chris Frontino, Sharon Butler, Judy Hall and Susan Gadwa; neonatal respiratory therapists Kim Wibben, Clyde Mori and Greg Moses; Chris Lombardi, manager of the NICU; Karol Norris, clinical nurse specialist; Sara Masur, occupational therapist; Dr. Robin Doroshaw, pediatric cardiologist; and Dr. Mel Marks, administrator of Miller Children's Hospital. Thanks also to Dr. Alan Boucher and Dr. L. Philippe Theriot, who helped pave the way. I am deeply grateful to the following families for their generosity of time and spirit, and their help and patience with my many questions: Robert and Amalia Allman, Kristine and Stuart Hawkshaw, Lisa Lee, Monique and Mark Hachigan, and Maricela and Enrique Leos. Finally, I wish to acknowledge the writings and research of a pioneer in neonatology, Dr. William A. Silverman, and, in particular, his book, *Retrolental Fibroplasia: A Modern Parable* (New York: Grune and Stratton, 1980), which contributed greatly to my understanding of the history and ethics of neonatology and the epidemic of blindness that struck more than ten thousand infants fifty years ago.

— Edward Humes
www.edwardhumes.com

PART I

NEW ARRIVALS

"The room even surgeons are afraid of"

1

Admission History and Physical:

Allman, BB

Day of Life: 1

Days in NICU: 1

Condition: . . . . Critical

Robert Allman races down the hospital hallway, following the plastic embossed signs leading him toward his son, a baby born far too soon, a frighteningly motionless child who had been swept from the delivery room inside the heated acrylic case of a premature-infant transporter, bound for something called the "Nick-you." That was how the nurses pronounced it, turning the acronym into words, confusing Robert until his stress-fogged mind pieced it together. Nick-you . . . NICU. Neonatal Intensive Care Unit.

How could he have forgotten that? They had told him about the Nick-you, showed it to him, readied him for it—though that brief tour seemed a lifetime ago, which in a way it was. His son's life had not yet begun back then. Now the baby was here. And everything was going to hell.

Robert thought he was prepared for this moment, but he wasn't, he realized, not even close. Both he and Amalia had been lulled by nine uneventful days of hospital bed rest, her leaking amniotic fluid and premature labor stopped in its tracks by powerful drugs. They were buying precious time, the doctors said. Every extra day in the womb meant the baby's survival chances would increase. Each day they held out without rushing to the delivery room, each day Amalia spent confined to bed twenty-three hours a day like some prisoner in solitary, meant two fewer days in the Nick-you for the baby, the doctors said. If they could somehow hold out for six weeks, they'd be home free: The dangers and uncertainties of premature birth would vanish like a nightmare at daybreak.

And it had looked for a time as if that might happen. Amalia Allman had been determined to keep that baby in, by sheer force of will if necessary. She had always been the strong one, Robert would say, the one who had grown up first and had helped him do the same. Whereas he would have gone stark raving mad, she had settled in with her books, her cross-stitching, his Game Boy, camped out for the long haul. When she had made it past the first forty-eight hours, a nurse had told her she was over the hump: Half the premature labor cases never made it to this point—she was doing great.

But today, day ten, out of nowhere, the contractions had kicked back in with a vengeance, excruciating and insistent, unstoppable this time despite the IVs, the breathing exercises, the prayers. The delivery had been awful. Despite the baby's half-normal size, his shoulders had been turned in such a way that he had gotten stuck. The neonatologist had stood poised at the foot of the operating table to receive him with a blue warming blanket in hand, exchanging worried glances with her nurse as the obstetrician struggled to extract the little boy. The fragile baby had been bruised from head to toe in the process, his head pulled into a frightening cone by the force of the vacuum extractor used to wrest him from the womb. He had cried, but just for a moment. Then the neonatal team had gone to work, the cries silenced by a plastic tube and the sudden, searing flow of pure oxygen down his small windpipe.

Now all Robert could think of were the stuffed animals he hadn't had time to buy, the baby's room that was nowhere near ready, the sheer normalcy of their shattered plans, all of it contrasted with the image of that tiny bruised baby—oh, God, he was so bruised—who hadn't cried or moved or even looked quite real as he entered the world. He and Amalia had barely gotten a look at him. Holding their son had been out of the question: He was headed to Baby ER.

Now Robert simply wants to find him, the vivid cartoon characters and nursery verse adorning the corridors of the children's hospital passing by in a surreal blur. "Go," Amalia had told him as they stitched her up, "I'll be fine. Just go. Stay with him." And so he dodges visitors and gurneys, desperate and helpless and alone, running toward his new son, toward the unknown.

2

Loud, bright and bristling with technology, Room 288 is the heart of the NICU, the starting point for the newest, the smallest and the sickest patients, the most "intensive" room in the five-room, seventy-one-bed Infant Special Care Unit at Miller Children's Hospital. The most extraordinary medicine happens here, practiced upon some of the most extraordinary patients there are, yet it is a place shrouded in mystery, closed off from view except for the doctors and nurses who love it and the parents who wish their children could be anywhere else but here.

Enter and find a room perpetually in motion. The neonatologists and their apprentices gather for rounds, a shuffling of feet and notepads, of last-minute phone calls and just one more hurried entry in a sick child's chart. Nurses are posted by their small patients, monitoring their progress, administering drugs, changing bandages—ever watchful for the slightest signs of distress or disease. RTs—respiratory therapists—move from baby to baby, adjusting ventilator pressures and oxygen flows, responding to alarms and looking for the mottled color or heaving chest of a baby approaching asphyxia. Lab techs come and go, drawing tiny blood samples from the babies' heels. Medical specialists from cardiology, ophthalmology, neurology and a host of other ologies perch on stools as they page through charts and scribble notes and recommendations. Other doctors perform treatments and even surgeries right in the room, many of them wearing magnifying binoculars, bent over their work like watchmakers, so small are their patients' organs and vessels. Pharmacists calculate medication dosages at bedside while nutritionists figure out the correct intravenous feeding solutions, walking a biochemical tightrope to balance the premature infants' delicate but volatile blood chemistry. Ultrasound technicians push unwieldy contraptions into position to capture ghostly images of tiny brains and hearts and kidneys, the organs swimming into and out of focus on small video screens as the techs move their magic wands over their patients. And everyone scurries to the other side of the room when a lead-aproned expert from radiology muscles her portable X-ray cart into position, shouts, "Shooting!" then fires up the machine. Whenever possible, the hospital comes to the babies rather than the other way around, which is a good thing, for the typical bumpy ride to radiology or cardiology might be fatal for these fragile patients. But as a result, the fifty-by-thirty-foot room at times seems ready to burst, an overpopulated aquarium, its fish swimming in all directions at once.

At the center of this activity are, of course, the babies, though they often seem dwarfed, even lost, amid the technology keeping them alive. Only twelve kids can fit in this room at any one time because of the enormous bulk of equipment tiny preemies and critically ill newborns require, along with the enormous manpower necessary to treat them: eight or more nurses, two respiratory therapists, an attending physician, a neonatal fellow and a medical resident. The room was designed for the equipment of the seventies, but nineties-era computers, monitors, ventilators and other space-hungry devices have taken over much of the white Formica counter space and open floor areas. Now the bodies and equipment barely fit, and walking (or running) without jostling the babies requires an almost balletic precision.

Each child lies inside an Isolette incubator, a clear acrylic rectangle with ample room for a half-sized premature baby, though the quarters become tight for the full-term eight-pounders. The tiny preemies who make up the bulk of the children in this room, many weighing less than two pounds, are displayed on cottony white bedding like wrinkled brown gems in a jewel case, bright jaundice-killing "bili lights" shining down on them like museum spotlights. Each Isolette's plastic casing and the baby inside sit atop a large blue-and-beige metal box on wheels, bristling with heating controls, humidifier settings and an array of sensors, plugs and conduits, the umbilici of technology. The incubators have portals of various sizes for admitting IV lines, wires, ventilator hoses and hands. The front panels flip down, and the bedding trays, which can lie flat or at an incline, slide in and out like kitchen cabinet drawers, allowing easy access to the patient inside—every incubator is, in essence, a miniature operating theater. The incubators are not soundproof, however; depending on the type of equipment in use, especially the ventilators and their various pumps and pistons, the interior of these lifesaving islands of machinery can actually be the noisiest places in the room. Oftentimes the nurses must put miniature ear protectors on the babies, bright orange, like airport baggage handlers', to keep them from being overwhelmed by their new environment or even deafened.

Room 288 is not only a place of continual motion. It is also a place perpetually filled with sound, the thrumming cacophony of an orchestra badly in need of a tune. There is the distinctive timpani chug of the oscillating ventilators hooked to the patients with the most fragile and damaged lungs, offset by the snare-drum whoosh and whisper of the conventional vents and the train-engine chug and rain-stick patter of another type of breathing machine, the high-frequency jet. Several times a minute, the high-pitched electronic bell of a cardiac monitor signals a heartbeat that is too slow or too fast. Newcomers to the unit jump each time these warnings sound, but the old hands know that the majority of them are false alarms caused by a baby's random kick or yawn that jogs the sensors. These alarms are often coupled with the soprano chime of pulse oximeter sensors signaling too much or too little oxygen saturation in the bloodstream—a type of warning less likely to be a false alarm and more likely to generate an immediate response from a nurse or respiratory therapist concerned about a baby's "sats."

Tenor and baritone bells signal a blood pressure drop or respiratory failure. In the background, there is a constant beat of electronic bleats emanating from Christmas tree–like formations of digital drug infusion pumps, hung by the dozen from chrome-plated poles throughout the unit and hooked into the babies by foot after foot of clear plastic tubes that wind around and inside the Isolettes, which have their own temperature and humidity alarm sounds. Overlaid on this mechanical din is the constant buzz of conversation among nurses, doctors and staff, some of it business, some of it social: the latest movie, the latest reason to rag on the hospital administration, the latest bit of unit gossip merging with talk of resuscitation, developmental delays and "Is it real?" inquiries about some alarm or other sounding in the unit. All of this is periodically drowned out by the cough of the cursed Stentofon, a wall-mounted speaker system that regularly bellows urgent requests for a neonatal team in the operating room, the women's hospital or the emergency room, with a sound quality only slightly less pleasing than the drive-through at Jack-in-the-Box, and a nasty habit of making the ordinary sound critical and the critical routine. And in the background, whenever the main entrance door to Room 288 opens, the timer-controlled faucets on the aluminum scrub sinks just outside the room add a metallic pounding to the clamor.

None of the noise, light and bustle is good for the hypersensitive systems of premature babies—just the opposite—but no one has yet figured out how to build a dark, silent intensive care room. It would be like trying to make flying safer by fashioning an airplane out of a Sherman tank. Theoretically, such a craft could survive any crash. But it would never get off the ground.

There is only one sound missing from this high-tech orchestra, one that should be most common in a nursery: the sound of babies crying. With oxygen-carrying endotracheal tubes eased down tiny throats and through vocal cords, and with infants sedated or placed in a drug-induced paralysis or just terribly weak, crying is rarely heard. And when it is, the sound startles the nurses and doctors more than any alarm, for crying is out of place here: A baby strong enough to cry is almost always too well for Room 288. There are four other rooms for babies who can cry—the intermediate care "step-down" rooms or one of the other less intensive sections of the NICU, to which babies are moved once they near wellness or at least discharge. The staff calls the least intensive area the "Fat Farm" because the major activity inside is eating and gaining weight (which is trickier than it sounds for a preemie, whose digestive system is more sluggish than a hospital bureaucracy). Room 288, though, that's for the new kids, the sick kids. Most of them *lose* weight in here.

Into this maelstrom come all new admissions to the NICU, most of them premature babies, all of them in critical condition. The tiniest preemies need months of care before they are ready to go home—usually around their mother's original due date, when they finally catch up to where they should have been all along. Other patients are in for a spectrum of ailments ranging from the minor to the harrowing: infections, jaundice, lung problems, heart conditions, birth defects or asphyxia. Most arrive fresh from the labor/delivery rooms on the other side of the medical center or from the adjacent operating rooms where cesarean sections are performed, sometimes at a moment's notice, an NICU team racing to gown up and take over the newborn as the surgeons cut. About a fourth of patients come via ambulance from other hospitals, wheeled in by special transport teams through the emergency room one floor directly below. And, on rare occasions, a panicked parent races up to the front desk with a sick infant clutched to breast, sometimes on their doctors' orders, sometimes appearing with no warning. Competition among hospitals for these children is fierce, but as the largest NICU in the area, Miller Children's gets the lion's share, treating about 1,100 babies a year. At any one time, there may be sixty to seventy babies here, making it one of the largest such units in the nation. The babies stay anywhere from three days to four months, with a few—particularly the kids with damaged lungs—lingering almost long enough for birthday cake. A few never leave.

The flow of children into the Miller Children's NICU is constant. There is a simple reason for this: One out of ten babies born in America is premature. One out of twelve newborns has a dangerously low birth weight. One out of every ten infants will need to stay in a place like Room 288, because of prematurity, birth defects, infection or all three. And these numbers are accelerating: More low-birth-weight babies were born at the end of the millennium than in any year past, which is one reason why America's infant mortality rate is an abysmal twenty-fifth in the world. It's also why the nation's network of 1,400 NICUs and 3,000 neonatologists is second to none: Supply follows demand. Neonatology, it seems, is a growth business, and likely to stay that way for the foreseeable future.

This is something most expectant parents understandably prefer not to think about, and something many hospitals (the ones with few or no neonatal capabilities) prefer to downplay. One reason for this silence is economic: Most hospitals and HMOs want to deliver babies in-house, with all their glorious billables, without investing in a full-service neonatal intensive care unit or paying to have neonatologists on duty around the clock. The market for delivering the nation's 4 million babies each year is among the most profitable in medicine's beleaguered economic picture (which is why costly emergency rooms—the first and sometimes only option for medical care for the uninsured—are being shuttered all over America, while new and remodeled labor/delivery departments are being minted all the time). Luring pregnant mothers is big business. Many hospitals market their luxurious birth suites and free HBO and gourmet meals while neglecting to mention that they have little to offer the one out of ten babies who ends up needing an NICU. Those children will have to waste precious minutes or hours being transported by ambulance, separated from parents and bumping through traffic instead of receiving lifesaving care right where they were born.

This high-stakes gamble pays off for 90 percent of families—most will never know what they missed or that they have rolled the dice with

their babies' lives, because the odds are with them. But those unfortunate 10 percent—and in America, that adds up to more than four hundred thousand babies a year—find out the hard way that some
hospitals boasting state-of-the-art facilities for delivering babies are not
so good at handling them once they're born. Forty thousand of these
babies will need long stretches of very intensive care. Yet many hospitals
delivering babies cannot put a breathing tube into an infant or provide
mechanical ventilation when a baby's lungs fail, and most lack the expertise to administer the gamut of lifesaving drugs that are routine in a
big, busy NICU—a Level III facility, to use the term neonatologists em-
ploy. Many hospitals with obstetrical wings may not have a pediatrician
in the building around the clock, much less a neonatologist, and those
that have them often have inexperienced medical residents working
largely unsupervised during the inconvenient late-night hours when
most babies seem to be born. A recent study of seriously ill babies born
in hospitals with large, full-service NICUs shows they have a 38 percent
better survival rate than sick children born in hospitals with small or
no neonatal programs.

Most expectant parents remain blissfully unaware of all this unless
the pregnancy happens to have been identified early on as high risk because of the mother's age, a medical condition, or a problem with the
developing baby. The rest do not find out if they chose their hospitals
well—or badly—until it is way too late to do anything about it. Which
is why so many small patients arrive in Room 288 via ambulance from
other hospitals with their parents pale and terrified in the car behind
them, unable to comprehend either their child's illness or why they
made the mistake of starting out at the wrong hospital in the first place.
Invariably, among the first words out of these parents' mouths—after
How is our baby?—is *Nobody told us.*

There is another, less obvious reason expectant parents are unaware
of this room: Even the outside doctors, nurses and medical students
who occasionally visit, work or train in the NICU find Room 288 a
daunting place. It takes a certain kind of person to make a career here;

those who take to it rarely seem to leave. The least senior nurse on the day shift has worked in this unit for twelve years; a few have been here as long as there has been an NICU in this hospital—twenty-five years, beginning when neonatology was itself still in its infancy. But others in the medical profession fear and detest the NICU, avoiding it whenever possible. Some do so out of grudging respect for the medicine practiced here or out of recognition of their own limitations. Others do it with a sneer.

"You know, some people in the hospital think all we have to do is flip 'em and feed 'em and watch 'em grow," says Donna Prochnow, an NICU nurse for seventeen years (and before that, a young mother whose son was treated in this room). Donna is repeating a familiar cliché heard from other medical disciplines, which tend to glorify surgeons and physicians who specialize in individual organs, rather than neonatology, which encompasses an entire organism. This is part of her stock lecture to the new nursing grad and NICU prospect she's orienting today. As she speaks, they wheel an infant into place after a trip to the CAT scan lab in the basement (one of the few tests that cannot come to the baby) and a respiratory therapist locks down the oxygen hoses with a high-pitched whistle of gas under pressure.

"There's a lot more to the NICU than that," Donna tells her new student. "This is life on the edge, my dear. Nowhere else do they have to weigh their patients by the gram instead of by the pound just to avoid a drug overdose. Nowhere else is the margin of error so small. This is the place to be—not for the money, not for the great hours. This is the place to be because it's *fun*."

Other nurses in the unit nod at these words. Like nurses everywhere, they have elevated complaining to an art form, but this unit is in their blood, an elite assignment for professionals who have become accustomed to working miracles, for bringing hope and life to a place where, just ten or fifteen years ago, tragedy seemed all too common. The neonatal nurses are the backbone of this place, filling an impossible job that is at once traffic cop, social worker, lifesaver, therapist, record keeper, undertaker and grief counselor rolled into one. The nurses here have unusual autonomy; they are empowered to make treatment decisions, to adjust oxygen settings, to double-check and even question the prescriptions and orders of their superiors, the physicians—an easing of the usually strict medical pecking order that is part of the fabric and mystique of this particular NICU and one of the reasons so many nurses make their careers here. Nurses in Room 288 are rarely assigned to more than two infants at once and often work one-on-one—a level of attention provided in few other places in the hospital, where managed care and yearly budget cuts have left nurses in short supply and adult patients pounding their call buzzers in frustration.

When you show up for a shift in Room 288, Donna tells the new nurse, you never know what the day will bring. Some people sky dive. Some climb mountains. In the NICU, they have their own way of challenging nature: bringing life to a place where, for 99.9 percent of human history, death has reigned supreme.

"But, you know, it's not for everyone," she adds, spotting the uncertain look on her student's face—a familiar expression, one that says this kid might not last a week here. Another nurse puts it this way: "You know what they say—this is the one room in the hospital even the *surgeons* are afraid of."

Dr. Arthur Strauss, medical director of the NICU, stands out in this blandly colored room of beiges and institutional blues like a splash of neon in his brightly colored Hawaiian print shirt. A gray cookie-duster mustache droops at the center of his long, craggy face, his head is topped by iron-colored waves, a stethoscope hangs around his neck. He rubs tired eyes and surveys his domain from his trademark cross-legged slouch in one of the unit's uncomfortable swivel chairs.

"Are we ready yet, Pure?" he asks the other doctor in the room, his voice and expression conveying the impatience his posture fails to communicate. "We're running late for rounds. Again." Then he makes his most frequent complaint, one regularly echoed by his colleagues in this medical era of unlimited bureaucracy and limited everything else: "We need to move along. I've got meetings all afternoon."

"Almost done, Doctor," answers the senior fellow, a pediatrician about to complete her three years of hands-on training in neonatology. Wearing surgical gown, mask and gloves and working intently, Dr. Purificacion Tumbaga does not look up from the new admission who is prone and sedated on a warming table in front of her: Baby Boy Allman. Pure is absorbed in the delicate task of inserting an IV line through the baby's badly bruised umbilical cord. She speaks distractedly: "Just a few more minutes."

Art grunts an okay and returns to scribbling in the chart of one of the more difficult patients in the unit. He knows Pure is one of the best fellows he's seen and that she'll run through the admission protocol for the new kid as fast as he could. Maybe faster.

Art is one of those smart, gruff, aloof-seeming physicians who tries to hide his kindness beneath a tendency to grumble and mutter—but who has been known to slip a twenty-dollar bill to a young mother so she can afford to buy a prescription for the preemie he is about to discharge. You don't often see docs reaching into their own wallets this way, but to Art, healing a child, then sending her home without everything she needs to thrive, is just plain wrong. He thinks no one is looking when he does this sort of thing, but the nurses see everything (and then, of course, tell everyone), and they love him for it. And so Art is beloved in the NICU both as a leader and as a target of good-natured torment from the nurses he has grown up with here for more than twenty years. This week it is his turn to preside over Room 288—the neonatologists rotate through the different rooms of the NICU, keeping fresh, avoiding burnout—and with that duty comes the privilege of running Morning Rounds. Most days the ritual of rounds moves to the back burner, crowded out by Code Blues, calls to the OR, new admissions. Today is no exception.

As Art looks at his patients' latest labs—all too many of them flagged as critical instead of within normal limits—he can see, out of the corner of his eye, a rumpled fax sitting on the counter. The document concerns the latest unwanted corporate takeover attempt of the NICU practice. Neonatology is good business these days—not only is prematurity on the rise, which guarantees a stream of patients, but insurers are far less likely to deny coverage for sick babies than for other, older patients, fearing negative publicity and a groundswell of support for more regulation. This means NICUs are among the most profitable departments in many hospitals, which is why they are being targeted by Wall Street medical conglomerates. The Long Beach NICU is a particularly inviting plum: well established, highly regarded, and with a long history of operating comfortably in the black.

Ever since 1994, when Art and his three partners wrested control of the NICU from their former mentor, a living legend who preceded them for eighteen years, they have found themselves swamped as much by the business of medicine as by the medicine itself. It used to be that technology, treatments and technique were the fastest-changing aspects of the profession. If you kept your skills up, you would succeed—you could be the best. Now such concerns seem increasingly irrelevant: It is the *economics* of medicine that are constantly changing at a dizzying pace, something to which Art's generation, trained in the seventies and eighties, had previously given little thought. Now one of the most popular subspecialties at medical school is an MBA. His residents may not be able to intubate a preemie the way he could when he was their age, but they sure can handle a spreadsheet. It irks Art, who at forty-seven suddenly feels like a dinosaur, struggling to keep up with evolution. "This is not what I signed up for," he complained morosely when his partner handed him the fax.

The medical director stretches, stifles a yawn. Neonatologists are almost always tired, given their horrendous hours, constant emergencies and regular stints on night call. In this hospital, they are among the only attending physicians who still cling to such hands-on medicine as weekly night call. Other parts of this hospital—and most other

NICUs—leave nights and holidays to the fellows and residents, the traditional scut workers of medicine, who make pennies on the dollar as they earn their licenses. Not in this NICU. One of the attending neonatologists is always here, twenty-four hours a day. This made for an especially grueling lifestyle until a year ago, when the four attendings who owned the practice handled everything. The long nights are fewer in number now that two former neonatal fellows who trained in the unit, Dr. Steve Cho and Dr. Leonel Guajardo, have joined the group, but ten- and twelve-hour workdays are still the norm.

Art looks over the patients in his care this day. The room is tough today. Ugly, Art thinks to himself: ugly because so few of the babies in here can be quickly healed, fattened up and sent home. Instead, an unusually high percentage of the current crop of patients is made up of long-term, chronically ill babies facing very uncertain futures. And though they often provide the most interesting cases, nothing is uglier to a neonatologist than a roomful of "chronics."

First, there are the triplets by the door, micropreemies weighing in at less than a pound and a half each at birth. The Lee boys are "twenty-four-weekers," born during the twenty-fourth week of pregnancy, rather than the forty weeks nature intended, and the odds for their survival are, at best, fifty-fifty. (Fifteen years ago, maybe ten, they would have had little to no chance at all—advances have come that fast and that far.) They look more like mummified old men than babies, for preemies at this stage of life have not yet formed subcutaneous fat. Their skin hangs loose on their twig limbs, a downy parchment that tears at a touch and retains neither heat nor moisture. A preemie can lose 20 percent of his body weight through evaporation alone, and these triplets don't have 20 percent to spare.

They are so immature, they lack the instincts to suck, to swallow, to cough, even to breathe. Their immune systems are so poor that a simple cold can kill. Their brains and nervous systems, geared to the wet, dark world of the womb, cannot yet handle the sensory overload of our world—the noise is jarring, the sights a bizarre blur, the gentlest of touches excruciatingly painful. Their lungs are a mess, demanding rivers of extra oxygen delivered at enormous pressures just to keep them from asphyxiating. To them, normal room air, with its meager 21 percent oxygen content, is like the rarefied atmosphere atop Everest. The Lee triplets need three times that, sometimes more. No organ or system in their bodies works properly, not even after three weeks of surgeries, antibiotics, transfusions and round-the-clock, one-on-one care. Even their circulatory system flows the wrong way, sending too much blood to the lungs, flooding them like a backed-up carburetor. This backflow is an illness only outside the womb—caused by an extra vessel that, before birth, serves as an efficient bypass for lungs that are not supposed to be breathing for another four months. The extra vessel withers away in full-term infants, but can linger dangerously in prema-ture babies. Caring for such micropreemies isn't about helping them along so much as it is about forcing their bodies to do things nature never intended.

Twenty-four-weekers exist at the outer boundary of medicine's ability to save premature children. Indeed, fetuses at this stage of devel-opment could be legally aborted in another part of the hospital. Every-one who works in the unit knows there is a grim calculus to all this: The difference between the bigger, heartier babies in the outlying rooms of the unit, the *growers* and the *feeders,* as the staff calls them, and the ba-bies in Room 288 amounts to little more than a few ounces and a few more precious days in the womb. A baby born at twenty-three weeks has more than a 90 percent chance of dying; after twenty-six weeks, the odds reverse, becoming 90 percent in favor of survival. It is that three-week range in between that is the diciest, the uncertain place these triplets occupy, the place where doctors and nurses and parents some-times ask, *How far can we go? How far should we go? How much is too much?*

Yet these little ones kick and yawn and wave their puny doll limbs in jerky, marionette motions, tugging ineffectually at the tangle of wires, hoses, sensor pads and IV lines covering them. The tiniest diapers the nurses can find are still ludicrously large for their kindling-sized legs and fat-free rumps, and the white cotton bandages covering their IV sites and livid surgical scars stand out in sharp relief to their bruised and yellow skin. Beneath all this technology, their essential human form is sometimes difficult to discern. Out of practical necessity, the babies are as cruelly naked and as exposed as trussed turkeys, displayed like specimens in their plastic-walled universes, and yet much of them is hidden from view by the machinery of medicine. Parents can spend months staring into an incubator as if into a crystal ball, yet have no idea what their child's face looks like.

The triplets' mother, Lisa Lee, is singing and praying by their bedsides as Art Strauss watches. Where others see infants wracked by pain and disability, she sees beauty, potential, a long-held dream fulfilled. "I think they're just sleeping," she says to a nurse, pointing to one comatose child, "and that soon they'll wake up and feel better." Her hope is unflagging, despite three difficult weeks of near-constant setbacks. She is forty-two, a woman so desperate to be a mother after thirteen years of failed attempts that she turned to aggressive fertility treatments. Perhaps too aggressive, Art thinks to himself. The treatments worked, but the mother did not count on one of the unadvertised shortcomings of fertility treatments: the increased likelihood that she would have multiple children, born prematurely and with a host of ailments. The triplets' monitors, multiple IVs and chugging ventilators tell the sad conclusion to this story: Without constant pumping and prodding with the best techniques and technology medicine can offer, they would die in seconds. Art now has to worry about a new mother who risks losing not one child but three. And who may be harboring very unrealistic expectations about their recovery.

Near the triplets is the five-month-old girl Art has been puzzling over this morning, Nikkol Hawkshaw. She was born with her intestines and part of her liver outside her body, a condition horrifying to behold though surprisingly correctable—but for the fact this was the worst such case seen here in thirty years. So far, nothing the doctors have tried is working for this baby. Her life is a daily exercise in agony. Her digestive system was put back into place surgically, but it cannot seem to accept food, even through the tube embedded directly in her stomach and designed to help even the most damaged babies keep food down. So bags of pale yellow intravenous fluid, a mix of protein, carbohydrates and lipids, keep her alive. But therein lies a trade-off typical of the NICU, the sort that at times makes neonatology seem like a stroll across quicksand: The baby's stomach, liver and intestines will atrophy and die unless she sheds her dependence on IV nourishment and begins to eat real food. If they cannot heal her gut soon and keep some real food inside her—"start feeds," in NICU parlance, a crucial milestone for every sick and premature baby—Nikkol will never recover. The girl's newlywed parents are alternately hopeful and desolated, grief-stricken and angry, grounded firmly in reality one day, gripped by wildly unrealistic expectations the next—what the nurses here call the NICU roller-coaster ride. One benign test result or an eyedropperful of diluted formula kept down starts the coaster on its uphill climb; the smallest of setbacks sends it crashing back to earth. Their feelings of helplessness have been magnified by the gastrointestinal specialists who consult for the NICU. They have been difficult to reach, too busy with their frantic and enormous multihospital practice to return phone calls, sending a different doctor to see Nikkol each time, who invariably tells the parents something different each time. They are furious at this, and this concerns the neonatologists, who don't like being dependent on outsiders, though in this unusual case, they have no choice. The Hawkshaws have no lives left outside their jobs and the hospital—no movies, no bike rides, no restaurant meals (except for the crumpled fast-food bags collecting in the backseats of their cars). They barely talk. The mother cries through the night. She can't eat. The stress of waiting is tearing them—and their marriage—apart.

Across from this child is an infant who would make the Gerber baby look anemic, a perfect, round, rosy cherub of a child, full-term, outwardly healthy—the sort of baby every other parent with an emaciated, struggling preemie in the NICU looks at with a furtive hunger, for they were denied such a child. But Jessica Jones is the daughter of a cocaine abuser whose drug of choice caused a catastrophic break in the placenta, depriving the baby of oxygen and destroying an otherwise healthy infant brain. Now Art is in the uncomfortable position of having to obtain consents and permissions from the same mother whose self-absorption and desire to self-anesthetize herself has consigned her baby to a joyless, sightless, vegetative existence. In a perfect world, many on the NICU staff say privately, the mother would be in jail and this child would be allowed to pass peacefully into death. In the real world, with all its quicksand choices, Art has to worry about the mother suing him and his hospital for doing too little for Jessica if she dies—or for doing too much if she lives. "Wrongful life" suits, they're called, the latest rage in the malpractice law: A hospital in Houston was just ordered to pay $43 million to the parents of a severely handicapped baby who was *saved* against their wishes.

Then there is little baby Miracle, the twenty-four-weeker who was supposed to be an abortion but whose mother went into premature labor before she could schedule the appointment. Because she was born twenty-four weeks after conception—four months premature—this micropreemie dwells at the extreme outer edge of viability, little more than halfway developed. Born any smaller or earlier, she would have had no chance. Yet Miracle is one of the healthiest kids in the room, confounding the odds and all expectations, though she is far from out of the woods yet.

Near Miracle lies the premature son of a surgeon who works in the medical center. His child's brain and reflexes are normal—for a twenty-eight-week-old embryo. The baby's system, geared to a life floating in amniotic fluid, has not yet fully developed the instinct for respiration. He forgets to breathe on an almost hourly basis. Every now and then, his respiration monitor line goes flat, alarms sound, and he has to be resuscitated—sometimes with a few pats on the back from his nurse to jar him back into breathing, sometimes with more drastic measures. He will eventually grow out of this, but his dad's medical knowledge has made the NICU experience infinitely more harrowing for all concerned. His wife finally had to tell him to stop describing to her all the worst-case scenarios he had heard of or she would lose her mind completely.

Next are twenty-five-weeker twins, born without prenatal care and, as a result, in enormous distress, with lung, blood pressure, heart and brain problems that otherwise might have been prevented. The nurses are furious with their mother, a homeless woman who admits to having used cocaine and cigarettes throughout her pregnancy—as she did with three previous children. The irony is that the drug-induced stress the babies suffered, even as it harmed their other organs, has helped their lungs—stress *in utero* can accelerate lung development and minimize the respiratory distress afflicting other preemies in the room. This by-product of addiction is one that the nurses are loath to discuss for fear of encouraging more maternal drug abuse—but there is no missing the fact that the NICU's drug babies, saddled as they are with a lifetime's worth of potential problems and handicaps, sometimes do seem to come off the ventilators faster than the kids whose mothers did everything right.

Next to the twins is a baby girl with a rare heart defect whose parents face a terrifying choice: They can try surgery to repair the missing portion of her heart. They can try for a high-risk transplant surgery should a new heart become available (though intact infant hearts are hard to come by). Or they can do nothing. None of these choices is easy. None has a guaranteed result, except for the third option, which is guaranteed to be fatal, though no one can say when. The shattered parents had no idea what was coming until the moment their daughter was born. Like their doctors, they had expected a perfectly healthy child right up until the time she was delivered. Then they watched her turn blue. The roller coaster hasn't stopped since.

Then there is little David Rios, the old-timer in the unit, a fuzzy-haired puzzle beloved by the nurses and respiratory therapists, whose heart, kidney and spine defects, missing lung and constant pain have left them with precious few options. He is always on the verge of a Code Blue, his breathing as unreliable as a drug addict's promise. No one can figure out how to get him off the ventilator, and this poses a deadly dilemma. Mechanical ventilators are lifesavers for preemies and other ill newborns, but they represent another of neonatology's quicksand trade-offs. Even as the vent keeps the baby alive, each mechanically induced breath damages the lung tissue. After a while, the damage can become irreparable. Which is why, in the NICU, getting babies *off* the ventilators is as much a priority as getting them on the machines in the first place.

David is old enough now to have forged bonds with staff members, to smile and look them in the eye and grab their fingers with surprising strength. He is smart and alert and angelic despite his twisted little body, and they are all desperate to help him. But so far, his condition has stymied their best efforts. All they know is that he is no closer to going home than when he arrived. And in the NICU, time does not heal all wounds: Beyond a certain point, the longer a baby stays here, the less likely he is to make it out. Some of his nurses have even wondered if it is time to discuss with the boy's immigrant parents a DNR—a "Do Not Resuscitate" order—so that David might be spared needless pain if his condition worsens. It was just lunchroom talk, something to think about down the line, but the normally laid-back Art reacted with uncharacteristic anger when he heard that it was being discussed.

"It's too soon for that sort of thinking!" he snapped. DNRs represent the end of the line in the NICU, an admission of failure. They are simple, one-page, fill-in-the-blanks forms that go at the front of the chart, and their innocuous appearance belies the reality behind them: an admission that all hope is lost. The NICU's medical director, who is also head of the hospital's bioethics committee, does not easily give up on a child, nor does he tolerate idle discussion of DNRs. He speaks passionately about this with the certainty that comes not just from twenty years in neonatology, but from a far more personal quarter: Art was a preemie himself.

"We've got a lot of options before we need to cross that bridge," he told the staff. "I want this talk of DNRs to stop. If it ever got back to the parents . . ."

He did not need to finish the sentence. Every nurse in the room knows that hope is the most precious commodity of all in the NICU— it keeps the parents coming day after day, enduring the worst times because they can hope for better. The staff is careful not to kindle unrealistic expectations, but they must be just as careful to avoid crushing hope. The talk of DNRs stops. For now.

Finally, next to David, there is the newcomer, Baby Boy Allman, three months premature, in distress, bruised badly from a difficult delivery, incapable of breathing on his own. He is an unknown quantity, slated for a battery of tests, assessments and measurements that are under way even as Pure continues to work on him, fresh from the delivery room, an oxygen tube threaded down his tiny throat.

And so, in this snapshot of time on this November day, there are twelve babies in Room 288, all of them sick, all of them challenging, none of them with fates easily predicted. Statistics suggest what is likely in each case, but in this room, more times than not, probabilities lose their meaning. No one who spends time here can say, with any degree of certainty, that one child has no hope while another hasn't a care in the world. The doctors and nurses have seen too many reversals of fortune, in both directions, to speak in absolutes. For good or ill, the NICU is a place of infinite possibility.

It will take three or four months before those possibilities narrow and the only question that really matters—*Will my baby be okay?*—can finally be answered with some confidence. That's how long it will take for the premature babies in the room to reach their original due dates and to catch up with nature. That's how long it will take for the treatments and surgeries and therapies to be concluded for the others, for the nurses and the doctors to become attached to their small charges and their families, for the bonds between parent and child to form and grow strong, for medicine's most cutting edge—a half million dollars' worth or more for the sickest among them—to work its miracles.

After all that, after all the science and heart and love and plain, unadulterated luck, eight of the babies in the room this day will go home in their car seats with their parents. And four will not.

3

ROBERT ALLMAN ROUNDS A CORNER AND FREEZES. SOMETHING has caught his eye: a large window through which he can see a row of babies lying in clear plastic cribs, swaddled and new to the world. They are crying and yawning and sleeping, untouched by tube, needle or machine. He is looking at the newborn nursery.

The cruelty is unintended, an accident of architecture: To get from the women's hospital at Long Beach Memorial Medical Center to the adjacent Miller Children's Hospital and its Neonatal Intensive Care Unit, the unlucky parents whose babies are housed there must first walk by the big picture windows of the regular nursery, where nine out of ten babies land after birth.

These windows are the first stop for proud new dads and grand-moms and big sisters who press themselves against the glass, waving balloons and stuffed animals, cooing and taking pictures, exchanging hugs of joy. Lamaze classes troop through, getting a peek at the prizes awaiting them. Expectant mothers in labor at the adjoining women's hospital are encouraged to walk by to see where their baby will be in a few hours, to take their minds off the pain of their contractions with a glimpse at the future. Big-brother and big-sister classes tromp by as well in an effort to soothe fears and dampen inevitable jealousies. It is the happiest place in the hospital. The screaming and stretching and blinking babies are irresistible, which is why you can always tell the NICU parents when they reach this point in the hallway: They're the only ones who stare straight ahead and walk faster, desperately trying to look anywhere but through that window at a world they have been denied.

It has been only a matter of days since Robert and Amalia Allman began touring community hospitals, looking through windows just like this one, trying to pick the best place to deliver their baby. The hospital in which they were now living hadn't even been on their shortlist—they had seen no need for a major medical center specializing in high-risk deliveries and ultra-low-birth-weight babies. They'd wanted comfortable rooms and a VCR and tasty snacks to get them through the long labor; their favored choice didn't even *have* an NICU. One tour included a raffle for the expectant parents whose business the hospital wanted, and the Allmans had won the grand prize: an infant car seat. "You must be a lucky charm!" Amalia had written the next day in the journal she was keeping for the baby. "Do you hear Daddy when he talks to you in the morning? He says 'Good morning' and 'See you tonight!' He bends over and talks to my belly. We love you and can't wait to see you." That journal entry, the last one Amalia had time to make before rushing to the hospital, her water broken three months too soon, had been captioned "91 Days to Go."

She had been ninety days off in her calculation.

Now they *had* seen their baby, all too briefly and far too soon, and the sight had not been like anything they had ever imagined. No one ever imagines being handed a baby like this, thin and pale and damaged, struggling for his very life. And the baby was not handed to them at all. He was taken away, their glance at him as quick as the flash of a camera, more afterimage than anything else, because in a blink he was gone, the beeping of his portable heart monitor fading as the neonatal team wheeled him down the hallway. It was a forlorn sound that made Robert want to cry.

All they had seen was that he was tiny. Wounded. Scary. Amalia was in tears. Robert felt as he had when he'd been a child and another kid had punched him in the stomach for no reason at all: utterly unprepared. He is a clothing and accessory designer; his job is to make people look like surfers, relaxed, effortlessly hip. His biggest worry three months ago was putting together enough collectibles from one of his great passions in life—the *Star Wars* movies—for him *and* his son to share (he settled things by buying two of every action figure), then putting on a brave face when Amalia told him no, they could not name their son "Jedi." Now he felt guilty, as if he should have been doing something else all those months, as if somehow he could have prevented this. It was crazy, untrue, he and Amalia had done everything the pregnancy books and the doctors had suggested, yet the thoughts kept coming: What sort of father, he kept wondering, lets this happen to his child?

As he passes it, Robert finds himself looking away from the "normal" nursery—he can't help thinking that word *normal,* and hating himself for it. He presses on. He is close now, the sign for the NICU just up ahead.

Part of his brain—the part that keeps on ticking in all of us with absurdly normal thoughts even during moments of crisis—records a simple mental note:

Next time, find a different route to the NICU. One that does not pass these windows.

4

THE MOST IMPRESSIVE, REWARDING, DISTRESSING, CHAOTIC, MESMERIZ-
ing aspect of the NICU—the choice of adjective varies moment by moment and room to room—is that it never stops. There is never just one
story unfolding, never just one life-and-death decision to make, never
just one expression of joy or sorrow or bewilderment. The NICU is not
a series of seventy-one patients being treated one after another like soldiers lined up at sick call, nor is it a tidy television show where the action pauses conveniently for commercial breaks and where entire life
stories can resolve themselves in forty-eight minutes. This place is
messy, more like a billiard game one second after the break, all balls in
motion, their end points still up for grabs. The room, the patients, the
treatments and the prognoses are in constant flux.

And so, while Robert Allman races to see his critically ill son and
Dr. Art Strauss waits to start rounds, and nurse Donna Prochnow
coaxes one of the Lee triplets to breathe at least a little bit longer, outside Room 288 two very different life-and-death dramas begin to un-
fold.

The first begins with a joke.

"Lupe's on tonight," Denise Callahan, the nurse coordinator this
shift, lets the nurses know. There are audible groans. "And you were
wondering why we've been so busy. These kids know she's comin'.
That's why they're all turning blue."

31

Dr. Guadalupe Padilla, one of the four partners who run the unit, had just poked her head into Room 288 for a quick word with Art. Lupe is the attending physician on call tonight; she'll work through the night and well into the morning, then may or may not go home. Now she shrugs and smiles at the familiar quip.

"What can I say?" There's genuine mirth in her voice—she's a woman who relishes banter. "It's all true."

There are stories about all the attendings—nurses cherish them, pass them on, maintaining an oral tradition for the unit. The Lupe stories are among the most gleefully retold. Unit legend has it that whenever the weekly schedule puts Lupe on call or in Room 288, admissions go up, emergencies multiply and the babies get sicker—a pattern even she agrees has held true since her days as a chief resident, when she earned the nickname "Angel of Death." The moniker, never spoken in earshot of parents or other outsiders, has nothing to do with her patients' outcomes, which are as good or better as any neonatologist in the business. She earned the "Angel" nickname because the staff feels worked to death whenever she's around. There are no studies to support this impression; it is utterly unscientific. But everyone who works here swears it's true.

"You know I'm good for the local economy," she says, then leans into the tiny coordinator's office, grabs a doughnut and heads back to her room.

Things just seem to happen more with Lupe around, this tall, imposing woman with flying dark hair and rumpled scrubs, who eschews makeup and nail polish and fashionable shoes as if they were infectious diseases, whose medical knowledge is encyclopedic but who never seems to know how to find her key ring or her beloved, essential, God-what-did-I-do-with-it-now PalmPilot scheduler. If she's monitoring the normal newborn nursery, more babies seem to need an NICU admission. If she's on nights, the babies seem to need resuscitation more often. Outlying hospitals call for more transport teams. The unit fills up like Los Angeles International Airport the day before Thanksgiving (which is good for the bottom line but bad for the nurses, who are sick of mandatory overtime and double shifts). One night, the unit got so crowded that a closet had to be converted to an extra patient care area. No one had to ask who was on call that night.

Given her reputation, Lupe somewhat proudly likes to proclaim herself the unit pessimist. Her glass-half-empty outlook, she says, is why she so readily errs on the side of admitting a baby to the NICU with even the mildest of symptoms, whereas some of her colleagues might take a wait-and-see attitude and let a child stay in the healthy newborn nursery for observation. Once an infant is admitted to the NICU, the minimum stay is usually three days, which is how long it takes to culture an infection—or to prove no infection is present. This is an eternity for parents who just want their babies home, so some neonatologists bend over backward to avoid that delay unless there is strong evidence that a newborn is sick. Not Lupe: She assumes the worst will befall any baby in question, admits the kid for the minimum three days, then hopes she is proven wrong—believing that seventy-two extra hours in the hospital is a small price to pay for a lifetime of peace of mind, both hers and the parents'.

Colleagues who know her best argue that this amounts not to pessimism but to an abiding (even optimistic) belief that *her* NICU is the best place in the world to be if you're a baby whose health is in jeopardy. The nurses put a more succinct spin on all this: Lupe, they say, is a control freak, a less than unique trait among physicians and one that Lupe happily admits to.

And so the Angel of Death legend has endured, the image of Lupe as a human tsunami spreading from the intimate confines of the unit to the hospital at large: When the latest crop of residents put on the annual roast of their mentors, the young doctor playing Lupe wore a hat with a giant black cloud attached. Whenever her character was about to speak, she would be paged to a medical emergency or some other disaster and would race offstage under her storm cloud, unable to complete even the briefest conversation. The skit was a showstopper, provoking laughs and hoots of recognition. Lupe's reaction was typical: "I've got to get one of those hats," she told her husband.

"What does she need the hat for?" Denise Callahan later quipped. "She's got a real storm cloud on her shoulder, everyone knows that."

As if in confirmation, the Stentofon barks to life. "We've got a crash C-section in OR-9," the voice in the wall-mounted speaker informs the room. "We've got decels and mec. They're cutting now."

In the women's hospital next door, Gillian Berger is already on the operating table, her abdomen about to be split wide open. It wasn't supposed to happen this way. Gillian is thirty-three, in perfect health. Until a few minutes ago, she and her husband, Harry, a food company executive, had enjoyed a textbook pregnancy. Every prenatal test had been normal, the ultrasound had looked great, the labor had progressed for hours without a hitch. They had every reason in the world to expect a textbook baby as well.

Then the numbers on the fetal heart monitor began to dip. The baby's heart was struggling, not with the normal periodic slowdowns brought on by contractions, but with an alarming condition called terminal bradycardia—prolonged drops below the newborn's (and soon-to-be-born's) normal minimum of one hundred beats per minute. A depressed heartbeat can prevent the brain and other vital organs from getting sufficient oxygen, causing permanent damage, even death. Or the heart problem might be symptomatic of some other life-threatening condition. There is just no way to tell without examining and treating the baby outside the womb. Getting the baby out—and, hopefully, ending the source of the distress—had suddenly become a matter of life and death, with no time to spare. The Bergers listened to a hurried explanation, their terror mounting, with the nurses prepping Gillian for surgery before the doctor had finished speaking. Then she was raced to the OR for an emergency cesarean section, her husband stunned, a camera meant to capture the joyous moment dangling forgotten from his wrist. And inside the NICU, the speaker on the wall sounded its harsh bleat:

Decels. Mec. They're cutting now.

"Decels" is an abbreviation for "decelerations," a reference to the alarming drops in the baby's heart rate. "Mec" is short for "meconium," the hard fecal matter that forms inside babies' intestines *in utero,* a substance stressed fetuses often pass into the amniotic fluid. It can then be inhaled, causing severe damage to the lungs. The neonatal team must use suction to remove the mec from the baby's mouth and throat and to treat the respiratory distress that inevitably results if some of the stuff still finds its way into the lungs. "Cutting now," as the words imply, means the preliminaries are over and the surgeon is going in. A neonatal team needs to gown up and get in there quickly, or the obstetrician will be standing there with a baby in hand and literally no one to hand her to.

This must be the most horrible and momentous event in the Bergers' lives, so it would no doubt bewilder them to learn that nothing about their personal nightmare seems particularly extraordinary or alarming for the NICU staff: decels and mec are seen on a daily basis, and treating them is usually easy. The staff is, of course, concerned and ready. But they know getting the baby out usually resolves the decels. The mec usually doesn't make its way below the vocal cords. And the team is used to hustling in at the last minute; there's nothing for them to do anyway until the baby is all the way out. If there were such a thing as a routine emergency, this would seem a good candidate. And so a first-year neonatal fellow, rather than an attending physician, goes over to handle the Berger delivery. She's done others that sounded a lot worse. No one gives it a second thought.

It takes less than a minute for the team to realize there is nothing routine at all about this emergency. Before she was even handed over by the obstetrician and wrapped in a blue receiving blanket, Baby Girl Berger began coding—hospitalspeak for dying, a variation of the venerable but descriptive medical euphemism, "Code Blue." Blood spews from the child's lungs when the fellow inserts a breathing tube and suction is applied. She is not breathing on her own. Her heart rate barely registers. When the fellow pulls the breathing tube back out to look for the cause of the bleeding, the child's heart thumps to a complete stop. While the nurse—the veteran P.M. shift coordinator, Martha Rivera—begins chest compressions, she asks one of the labor/delivery nurses to call the NICU: "Ask for one of the attendings. Stat."

Two minutes later, Lupe Padilla pushes into the room and takes in the scene: the baby in full code, the resuscitation under way, the respiratory therapist, a huge man named Greg Moses, moving gracefully in the tight quarters, "bagging" the child with his hand-pumped ventilator. The anesthesiologist who worked on the mother had to come over and help the neonatal fellow squeeze the breathing tube back into place, but he gives way when Lupe arrives. The sense of relief is palpable. It is for moments like this that Lupe has trained for ten years.

She says calmly, "Okay, whattawe got?"

"Pulmonary hemorrhage," the fellow says gravely. Lupe nods, thinking, *Damn. Why did it have to be that?* Bleeding from the lungs, she knows, is one of the most devastating ailments the NICU faces, because there is no way to physically repair the bleeding vessels inside the lung, and because it can destroy a life more quickly than virtually any other trauma, as the baby literally drowns in her own blood. Something must have gone badly wrong during the last hours of Gillian Berger's pregnancy—an infection, a blood pressure problem, something—and this is the result.

"They said it was mec, but there's no mec," Greg adds. "Just blood." He pauses in his administration of pure oxygen and uses his suction hose. The clear plastic tubing turns bright red once again.

"There's no heart rate, no respiration," Martha says grimly. "She's been down now for"—a glance to the clock—"three minutes."

"Okay, let's see what we have here," Lupe says, her gloved hands a blur over the child as she goes to work, her normally expressive voice now a careful monotone. As she speaks, she removes the breathing tube, then peers inside with her laryngoscope, a metal-handled, hammer-sized tool capped by a light and a dull, flat blade that can be thrust down a baby's throat. Lupe must push aside the tongue with the blade so she can visualize the vocal cords, finding a pathway for placing a breathing tube down the throat, past the larynx and into the trachea, so that the oxygen can be pumped at high pressure directly into the lungs. Intubating such a child—maneuvering the thin plastic endotracheal tube into a windpipe the diameter of a number-two pencil—at high speed, in a crisis, requires the finesse of a brain surgeon, particularly when copious amounts of blood are flowing, blocking the view. The residents watch in awe when their mentors do this without breaking a sweat.

"Okay, I'm in," she says after a few seconds. "Let's have a dose of epi, please."

A small amount of epinephrine is poured from a vial into the baby's breathing tube and blown into her lungs. Epi is one of the standard "code drugs" the team always brings to a transport or delivery—just in case. It is primarily a heart stimulant, but it also constricts blood vessels, a quality Lupe hopes will stanch the flow of blood from the baby's lungs as well as jolt the heart. At the same time, she quickly threads an IV line into the stump of the umbilical cord still attached to the baby, the quickest way to administer more code drugs. During codes, Lupe always goes for the gaping mouth of the single vein in the umbilical cord, an easy target compared to the two small and sometimes stubborn arteries in the cord. (Of course, "gaping" is a relative term: To a neonatologist, who thinks three-pound babies are huge, a "gaping" opening is about the diameter of a standard toothpick.) Lupe places the line in less than a minute. All the while, Martha keeps performing compressions, using a delicate touch and two fingers of one hand, while Greg continues to "bag" the baby, trying to substitute external force for what the baby's internal organs are supposed to be doing. Squeeze a chest and heart that are not moving, fill and empty lungs that are not breathing—and maybe there is still a chance.

"Another dose of epi, please." This one goes into the umbilical line, straight to the heart. The baby is still not responding; the sense of urgency mounts with each passing second as the odds of saving her slip away with each tick of the clock.

Baby Girl Berger is a pretty baby, Lupe can see. Looks perfect, chubby and bald. Lupe likes the bald babies. By all rights, this kid should be crying a hearty cry and lying on top of Mom's belly right now. She's a sucker-punch kid—the sort of baby everyone expected to be fine, who should be fine, but who crashes for no good reason. Beneath the streaks of amniotic fluid, blood and vernix—a thick, white, pasty substance that protects a fetus's skin; nature's cold cream, the nurses call it—the infant's flesh looks gray instead of healthy pink. Her limbs lay flaccid, splayed out limply like a carelessly positioned doll's. *This is an ugly one,* Lupe thinks. *This is not good.* Years ago, she backed out of a fellowship in pediatric intensive care because she could not bear the emotional toll of having to deal with older children dying, of seeing a five-year-old who had a wonderful life one day but was brain-dead the next because no one had seen him at the bottom of the swimming pool until it was too late. She had resigned from her fellowship after five months, telling her mentors she could not deal with it, and she had turned to neonatology, where a world of preemies and other babies who had no prior lives or bonds or expectations or crayoned pictures of Mom and Dad were somehow easier to take. Except for the sucker-punch cases, the full-term babies who look perfect—and their parents, who had expected to take them home in a matter of hours. Babies like this one evoke the same awful, sad feelings. They made her want to hug her own daughter.

But Lupe is the consummate professional. Her voice betrays no emotion and grows calmer with every order. Her requests grow even more polite, almost formal. "Thank you very much," she says after each urgent order is met. Later she explains this method of dealing with emergencies: "It's a way of exerting control over an out-of-control situation, a certain tone of voice. You get super, super polite. Sometimes, it's all we have."

At the root of Lupe's medical philosophy is an almost primal fear of making a mistake, a fear she embraces and makes use of every day. *Fear is your friend,* her mentor in the neonatal unit told her sixteen years ago during her residency, before she realized what she was getting into— before she knew enough to be afraid. *Fear keeps you honest, keeps you checking yourself. When you walk in this unit and feel no fear, it's time to go find a new job.*

Good advice, advice that goes to the heart of the way a doctor walks into a room and looks at a patient—and herself—is not easy to come by. These words stuck with Lupe: In every emergency, admission and delivery, each time she reviews a chart, peers over a resident's shoulder or dictates a History and Physical report, she remembers her mentor's warning. And she tries to remember her fear, rather than her confidence in herself, in her experience, and in all those machines, imagers and other devices that have made the hands-on physical exam a dying art—a trend she and her colleagues fight each day, even if some of the residents seem to consider touching their patients only slightly more advanced than the therapeutic use of leeches. Echocardiograms are wonderful tools, Lupe says, but I want to listen to every heartbeat with my own ears. She memorizes the most distinctive heart murmurs like ditties, then hums them back at the residents, asking them what some rasp or whisper or minuscule skip in an infant heart might mean. She questions herself even more rigorously, mostly in her head but sometimes out loud: Did I prescribe the right dose? Did I choose the right med? Was my diagnosis correct? Shouldn't I order another ultrasound or X ray just to be sure?

Whatever might be going on inside her head, few figures in the NICU inspire more hope in parents and confidence in staff than Guadalupe Padilla. Families find comfort in her easy, relaxed manner, the way she seems to relate with anyone who walks into the room. Is the father of one baby in her care a recent immigrant from a small town outside Guadalajara? There's Lupe speaking to him in Spanish and saying, "What a coincidence, that's the same town where my parents grew up." Has the mother of the baby in the neighboring incubator just returned from vacationing in the Caribbean? There's Lupe swapping cruise-ship horror stories with her: "All you do on those cruises is eat. Nothing in my suitcase fit me by the time we got to port."

So it goes with the oldest daughter of Mexican immigrants, who raised their children on L.A.'s affluent West Side, sending all eight off to college and professional careers (though Lupe's father, something of a Renaissance man himself, wanted his sometimes argumentative daughter to be a lawyer, not a doctor). Lupe bridges culture, class, language effortlessly. And, almost magically, her conversations with parents slip from personal chitchat to the fine points of abdominal surgery or treatment for respiratory distress, and suddenly Mom and Dad find the daunting medical talk less threatening. They are not speaking to a distant, authoritarian physician but to someone with whom they share common ground, who vacations in the same places or shares the same roots. With the staff, she is different but no less inspiring: She is a relentless nag, staying on top of every detail, even if it means fiddling with the dials herself instead of having a technician do it, because Lupe wants things just the way she wants them. "It's that control freak thing," she says apologetically, then continues whatever it was she was doing. The nurses and respiratory therapists sometimes get irritated by this, but one thing is certain: They never have to worry that they are being left too much on their own when Lupe is around. Everyone was glad to see her walk into the room and take charge as Baby Girl Berger crashed.

Still, for all her abilities, her calm, her take-charge manner, nothing is working at the moment. Four minutes have passed since the code began, and there is no heart rate, no respiration. Nothing.

"Let's have some bicarb, please," Lupe says. "Four mEqs." A needle with an infant-sized dose of sodium bicarbonate is emptied into the umbilical line. Bicarb counters the acids building up in the baby's blood—a dangerous by-product of poor circulation and no breathing. It also helps the epinephrine do its job. Albumin is pushed through the catheter next to replace the volume of lost blood, then dextrose—a shot of sugar to improve circulation and brain function—followed by another dose of epi. And another. The kid should be turning handsprings from these drugs by now, but still there is no response.

It has been five minutes since the baby was delivered, though it seems much longer. Lupe makes a mental note of the baby's five-minute Apgar score, a one-to-ten scale used to assess the physical reactions, vital signs and neurological state of a newborn (named for its inventor, a pioneering neonatologist named Virginia Apgar). Points are awarded for the strength of the baby's heartbeat, cry, respiration, color, reaction to stimuli. The scoring is done at one minute of life, then five minutes of life. If there's a problem, it continues at five-minute intervals until the score—and the baby—are stable. An average healthy newborn usually scores a nine or eight. No one gets a ten, the nurses say, except the children of obstetricians and neonatologists. Anything below a five indicates a problem.

Baby Girl Berger's one-minute Apgar was four.

Her five-minute Apgar, Lupe notes, is zero.

Zero means no heartbeat, no respiration, no movement. No life.

"Hello, baby, you're out," Lupe cajoles the still child. Baby Girl Berger's skin is no longer gray but chalky white, bloodless, waxy beneath the glare of the OR lights. Lupe peels back one of the eyelids, looking to see if the baby's pupils are wide open and nonreactive to light, a sure sign of massive brain damage. She smiles grimly, finding one encouraging thing to report: "No, they're not blown."

In the center of the room, the obstetrician, her assistant and the nurses are sewing their patient up, their tension dissipated. They are chatting, laughing, relaxed. For them, the drama is over. The total disconnect between the birthing team at center stage and the neonatal team crowded in one corner of the OR is disconcerting, as if they weren't in the same room. The OB looks up from her work and casually asks Lupe, "So how's the baby doing?" For her the emergency is done, and you can hear the lack of concern in her voice, unaware of the life-and-death struggle occurring only six feet away.

Lupe remains silent and shoots a look at the OB. Lupe doesn't know if the mother is awake or not and hesitates to say what she is thinking, which is, *We're losing this baby. And if we don't lose her, there may not be much left to take home.* Instead, she simply says, in a voice that sounds almost unconcerned, "We'll be right with you," then returns to work, asking another neonatal nurse, who has come to provide backup and is standing outside the OR door, to draw still more epi. The supply brought for the delivery has been exhausted. Blood is ordered from the blood bank, more bicarb is administered. Greg sucks more crimson liquid from the baby's lungs. Martha continues her compressions. "God, she feels cold," Lupe says, the baby's skin icy beneath her touch, even through the latex gloves. Baby Girl Berger is now ten minutes old. Her Apgar score is still zero.

When the official code report is filed in the chart the next day, her condition at this point will be termed "severe neonatal depression." But physiologically speaking, she is dead. The effects of lengthy periods without respiration and heartbeat are known to everyone in the room: The vital organs, beginning with the brain and progressing to the heart, lungs and kidneys, start to die. If enough of the brain is destroyed, the baby can suffer from cerebral palsy, developmental delays, paralysis, blindness and worse—assuming the child can be resuscitated at all. None of these are givens; they are merely possibilities that become probabilities with each passing minute. Lupe's efforts are not pointless, however, because babies, particularly full-term, full-sized, outwardly normal ones like Baby Girl Berger, are remarkably resilient. They can recover from insults that would destroy an adult. Still, there is a limit. Time is running out.

They reach the twelve-minute mark, twelve minutes without breathing, without a heartbeat—a very long time. If Martha's compressions are just right, if the lungs are working and the blood is still being oxygenated and if that blood gets to the brain and the other vital organs despite the lack of a working heart, it's still possible she can make it. A lot of "ifs," Lupe knows, which is why she is beginning to wonder when she should call the code. At fifteen minutes? They can't keep flogging this poor child forever. Calling the code means bringing the efforts to revive Baby Girl Berger to a halt. Lupe will look at the clock and pronounce the time of death, and one of the nurses will dutifully write it down, then they will all stand there and stare, dreading what comes next—with the mother under a surgical drape just six feet away, her belly still big from the child just taken from her.

"Come on, come on, you can do it," Lupe urges the child. It is the first time anything resembling urgency has crept into her voice. Then, resuming her excruciatingly calm tone, she asks for a sixth and final dose of epi, please. This one is for the breathing tube again, like the first, a slam to the bleeding lungs and the idle heart, a jolt of liquid electricity. In it goes, and Martha stops her compressions. She and Greg and Lupe bend over the motionless child, searching for a response. For a moment, it seems, all the people in the room hold their breath, an eerie, silent pause.

5

ROBERT ALLMAN SEES A PAIR OF HEAVY WOODEN DOORS, OVER WHICH hangs a sign, "Infant Special Care," and another that says "NICU." Suddenly, his feet feel heavy. This is the place he has been rushing toward, but now he feels a strange reluctance to enter, knowing that the threshold represents a point of no return, where any lingering fantasies of a miraculously healthy baby will be banished for good. A tall blond nurse wearing flowered scrubs is painting turkeys and cornucopias on the unit windows for Thanksgiving. She notices Robert's distress and lowers her brush. "Was your baby just admitted to the NICU?"

It wasn't really a question. There is no mistaking the expression on the faces of new parents arriving at the unit for the first time. Robert nods. "I'm looking for my son."

"Through the doors, check in at the desk, then you'll have to scrub up." The nurse speaks in the measured tones that the NICU staff always uses with newly arrived parents, who find it hard to process and retain even the simplest instructions—understandable under the circumstances. "And take a deep breath. Your baby's in the best place he can be."

Robert steels himself and walks through the doors. He finds himself in a short hallway with large nurseries on either side. At the other end of the hallway is a large counter made of dark simulated wood and, beyond that, a door leading to yet another nursery of some sort. Nurses, doctors and other people are moving around him with purpose, squeezing past him as he stands and gawks in front of the entrance. The most surprising thing is the noise in this hallway, unexpectedly loud and diverse. The hollow pounding of water streaming into scrub sinks the size of bathtubs dominates everything. This watery drumbeat competes with a nurse rattling around in a freezer filled with bags of breast milk. She is talking to another nurse about having to come in at 3 A.M. instead of her usual seven o'clock starting time because the unit is so full and busy. "It's getting so I'm afraid to pick up the phone," she's saying, a complaint so mundane and universal, it almost makes Robert smile. Slouching in an orange plastic seat at a white Formica counter, a girl in a hospital gown who looks all of fourteen answers questions for a young doctor in scrubs, who wants to know how many *other* children she has and whether they, too, were born positive for cocaine.

To Robert's immediate right, is a small room that resembles a telephone booth, with a sign that says "Dictation: Physicians Only." Through the thick glass, he can barely hear the muffled sounds of a man in sport clothes with a stethoscope around his neck, speaking incredibly fast, medical-sounding terms Robert does not begin to understand—rule out sepsis, gentamicin, head ultrasound—drifting out in singsong snatches. One of the new attending physicians is dictating an H and P—the admission History and Physical. This two-page report is written up each time a baby is admitted to the unit, the first in a sheaf of papers that will fill each baby's chart, which in the NICU is not a chart at all but a thick loose-leaf binder crammed with nurses' observations, test results, progress notes and photographs. He doesn't know it yet, but Robert is about to become addicted to deciphering the arcane language of this chart, for it will represent a tangible summary of his son's short life.

From this spot just inside the unit, Robert can see into several of the NICU rooms, though not Room 288, where his son is. That room is straight ahead, past the front desk and the glorified closet that is the nurse coordinator's office. But he can see more than enough from this vantage point unit to know he is entering a world for which he is ill prepared. He takes a deep breath and walks on rubbery legs to the front desk. "I'm here to see my son," he says. "Allman."

The unit secretary verifies that Baby Boy Allman has indeed just been admitted and explains the three-minute scrub-up ritual to Robert: "Go to the sink, push the silver button, keep washing up to your elbows until the yellow light turns green, dry off with the paper towels, then we'll take you in to see your baby."

Robert walks to the sink. There are four faucets, four silver buttons. He pushes one and, with a heavy mechanical thump, water begins streaming out. He tears open the green-and-white wrapper of a surgical scrub sponge, dribbles liquid soap onto it from a hand-cranked dispenser mounted on the wall, and gets to work, the soap and bristles and forceful spray of water turning his pale hands pink as he studies a diagram that shows the proper technique for washing. A sign tells him to remove his wristwatch and rings and any coat or jacket with sleeves, and to wash for three whole minutes, no cutting corners. The message is repeated in Spanish.

Jo Ann Elkins, the secretary, watches to make sure he is following instructions. More than any drug, surgery or therapy, she knows, those sinks are the single best disease prevention mechanism in the hospital. Sometimes, though, seeing the stricken expressions of the parents who only want to rush in to their babies, she feels more like a grade school teacher ordering her students to detention than the guardian of sterility in the NICU. Satisfied that Robert is doing a proper job of scrubbing up, she offers him an encouraging "That's the way." She knows three minutes is barely a blink of an eye in a hospital, where people wait for hours for everything. But when you're standing at that sink, waiting to enter the NICU for the first time, desperate to see your baby, those three minutes are a lifetime.

6

THE SUCKER PUNCHES ARE THE MOST GRUELING CASES FOR THE NICU.
Preemies, birth defects, developmental problems often come with advance warning. Mothers and fathers—and caregivers—have time to
prepare themselves for the uncertainty and pain to come. Sometimes.

With a sudden crash, however, the baby is usually full-term, outwardly beautiful. The parents had every reason to expect a perfect
child, and why shouldn't they? Didn't every doctor and lab test say it
was so? Wasn't that the deal? If they did everything they were supposed
to do—the doctor visits, the healthy food, the swearing off of coffee
and wine and diet soda and any other guilty pleasures—then they
would get to take home a healthy baby, right? Sometimes when the
crash begins and the neonatal team leaps into action, Dad is standing
there thunderstruck, unable to grasp the sudden tidal change in for-
tunes, his wife terrified and asking, "What's happening? What's wrong
with my baby?" The question hangs in the air unanswered. The husband is guided to a spot near his wife's head, so he can comfort her. And
where he will not have to look at what is about to happen.

This is how it is with the Bergers. And, in a very different sort of
way and a very different setting, this is how it is with Baby Boy Bernard.

Sammy Bernard is in Room 276, the NICU's intermediate room,
where attending physician Jose Perez is speaking gently with his young
mother, Susan. She is in tears.

Before them, her two-day-old baby lies inside an incubator, his head beneath a hard plastic oxygen hood nicknamed a "cake cover" because of its shape. The baby is not in crisis at the moment, nothing like the scene in OR-9, just a one-minute walk away. Yet he is worse off than Baby Girl Berger, who still has a chance. Sammy Bernard has none.

The child has Trisomy 13, a rare genetic syndrome that usually leads to miscarriage, but not always. About once in every twelve thousand births, a child is delivered alive with Trisomy 13. There is no cure, no treatment, no getting better. No hope.

Babies with Trisomy 13 have a third thirteenth chromosome; no one knows why it appears or how it wreaks the havoc it does on the human organism. It is the worst of the trisomy disorders (much nastier than the more common Trisomy 21, better known as Down Syndrome). The flaw in the genetic structure of these children causes terrible deformities: Sammy has microcephaly, a sloping forehead, closed fontanelles (the soft spots on an infant's head, normally open, that allow cranial and brain growth), a cleft lip, extensive heart defects, an extra toe on one foot, a simian crease on the palms of his hands, a hole at the base of his spine. There are other assorted abnormalities. The worst are the severe brain defects and profound mental retardation that always accompany Trisomy 13. This child will never develop mentally, never recognize his mother, never communicate or understand the images and sounds that his eyes and ears receive but cannot process. The higher brain functions simply aren't there—there is no capacity for memory, for dreams, for pleasure. Half of all babies afflicted with this syndrome die in the first months; by the end of a year, nine out of ten are dead, a long and painful march through uncharted territory for their families.

Dr. Jose Perez, the NICU's most fervent optimist, whose remarkable life includes arriving in America as a Cuban refugee, growing up in an orphanage, attending one of the nation's most exclusive prep schools, and establishing a stellar medical career, does not like Trisomy 13. It is one of the few cases in which he can offer a parent nothing but hopelessness, and Jose does not like to rob a parent of hope. He tells the nurses in the unit always to find something positive to talk about, no matter how bad things get. His entire medical philosophy—indeed, his entire life—is built on an almost religious belief in hope.

"Isn't there anything you can do?" the young mother wants to know. "An operation or something?"

She is only twenty, utterly unprepared for this terrible blow. Prenatal blood tests are not one hundred percent accurate; hers failed to detect the genetic abnormality, and because she was young and healthy, no other prenatal testing that might have revealed her baby's condition was called for. At first it was hard for her even to look at her child. Now, though, she is desperate for something to hold on to, anxious for an admission that there might have been a mistake somewhere and that her son has a small sliver of hope.

"I'm afraid there is nothing we can do for Sammy but keep him comfortable," Jose says wistfully. He rubs his salt-and-pepper beard, a small man in casually elegant attire. Most times he has an easy smile, a way of connecting with families that has made him one of the nurses' favorites. Today, though, there is nothing to smile about. He must have a neonatologist's least favorite conversation with a parent, a conversation about dying. "What we really need to consider," he begins, "is what's best for him—and for you."

Jose's voice is kind, patient, fatherly. He is in every way the opposite of Lupe's Calamity Jane persona. When Jose is on call, everyone sleeps. Admissions go down. The Stentofon might as well be disconnected. Stories of Jose's tranquil influence are, of course, nothing more than NICU legend again, as unscientific as they are accepted as gospel truth.

Jose's serenity makes him a master of such difficult moments, even as they pain him. This quality is hard earned, the legacy of a child who survived difficult times himself and who earned everything good in his life. He was born in 1949 in a small town outside Havana during the turbulent years preceding Fidel Castro's rise to power. Thirteen years later, he came to America alone and frightened, one small player in a massive smuggling operation whose cargo was not contraband but children. Operation Pedro Pan, as the project came to be known, joined the Catholic Church in Miami, the CIA, and the State Department with Cubans who opposed Communist rule.

More than fourteen thousand Cuban children were sent to the United States in the early sixties, ostensibly for family visits but with no real intention of returning to their homes. Jose's parents, like others who turned to Operation Pedro Pan for deliverance, wanted their son raised free of communism and safe from the civil war they expected would quickly depose Castro's regime. Jose's parents told him they would be together again in a matter of months, just as soon as Cuba was liberated.

But months turned into years, and children like Jose were relegated to a lonely, uncertain existence separated from their families by ninety miles of ocean—and the much larger barrier of the Cold War. Fidel Castro's staying power exceeded his opponents' wildest imaginings. Like so many other children of Pedro Pan, Jose found himself penniless and cut off from his loved ones by blockades and missile crises, his care entrusted to the church, which had agreed to look after the dispossessed Cuban children.

The diminutive thirteen-year-old with an indefatigable sense of humor first landed in a church-run boys' camp in Florida. As one of the older refugees, he became a genial ringleader for the other dispossessed children, refusing to complain or cry in front of the younger ones, vowing to suck up his pain and put on a carefree face for their sake. Next year, he would promise the other kids, we'll all be on the beach laughing about this. Someday, he'd predict, he would be a great doctor and all the refugees could be his patients. Only when he was in the shower, completely alone, did his willpower crack, did he break down and weep.

Later, Jose was shipped to an exclusive prep school in Delaware. The church had found him a fabulous school, but he arrived with no preparation. The Cuban country boy with no English and no money was supposed to fit in with children named du Pont who arrived at school in limousines. He had just his few paltry belongings and an old photo of his parents. He couldn't read the form that explained how to get a lock for his locker, so he carried everything with him from class to class. It took him six months to teach himself enough English to get by, a process he did not realize was occurring until he found one day he could understand what was being said in his science class and he suddenly realized he could think in his new language.

After two years, many children were reunited with their families during a temporary thaw in Cuban-American relations and a brief easing of travel restrictions. But Jose remained alone, his parents unable to get permission to leave. He and a few of the remaining refugees ended up in an orphanage in Lincoln, Nebraska, where subzero winters greeted a child of the tropics who had never seen snow in his life.

In 1966, during another political thaw, Jose's parents finally had a shot at leaving Cuba. It fell to their teenage son to write the State Department and arrange for the all-important visas, more precious than gold. He must have written the letter a hundred times in his head. This time, the application went through, and his parents finally came to the United States.

There is no mystery where Jose's sunny outlook on life comes from. His mother, a high school math teacher in Cuba, soon found work at a college in the states—as a janitor. When she wrote home, she cheerfully informed her proud relatives only that "I have a job at the university." His father, who had owned his own small store, found similar custodial work, and each of them took a different shift so one could always be at home to care for Jose's developmentally disabled younger brother. They soon went on to better jobs, but always worked hard and long hours. Jose, who became a straight-A student once he mastered his new language, turned down a scholarship to the prestigious University of California–Los Angeles in favor of Los Angeles City College so he could hold down a forty-hour-a-week job at a bank to help support his family while earning his degree.

He chose to study engineering, not because he loved it but because he felt it would lead to a lucrative career in fairly short order. These were boom times for California's aerospace and defense industries, and engineers were in great demand.

But his parents surprised him. They had not forgotten a young Cuban boy's dream of being a doctor, and they told him he had made enough sacrifices. They wanted him to follow his heart and go into medicine, even if it meant many more years in school with little income. They'd manage somehow. "You've earned this," his mother said proudly. When he arrived at the University of California–San Francisco med school, fate dealt him one more twist: his classmate, and later, best friend and fellow resident, was another child of Pedro Pan.

Today, when asked about his harrowing past, Jose will shrug and smile in a sort of elfin way, minimizing the bad times, saying his parents had been right to do what they did, that everything worked out, that he has, in fact, led a life blessed by good fortune. He has a wife and children he loves, a country he loves, a career better than any he could imagine, working with some of the best in his field. "How could I not be optimistic?" he asks when some of the nurses chide him for being too sunny at times. "I'm the luckiest person I know."

But not even the unit's most optimistic attending can change things for Sammy Bernard. There is no happy spin for Trisomy 13. They can relieve his pain while waiting for nature to take its inevitable course, Jose tells Sammy's mother, but that is all. And it is here, he says, that Susan Bernard can help her child. Should Sammy's heart or breathing stop, she could give Jose permission to withhold treatment, to instruct the NICU staff not to resuscitate. Eventually, this crossroads will be reached, and when it is, they need to be ready. They need her to sign a DNR. To spare Sammy needless and futile pain.

An unmistakable look steals across the faces of parents in the NICU as they absorb, for the first time, the certainty that their child is going to die. It is different from the expressions of fear and confusion so common here, different from the look of angry disbelief that often falls into place when the subject of death is first broached. This singular expression appears only after the inevitable protests and questions are exhausted: *Are you sure? Aren't there more tests we can do? Can't you operate? Shouldn't I get a second opinion?* Sometimes it takes minutes, sometimes hours, sometimes days, but when there are no more questions to ask and no more answers to be given, that look falls across the faces of mothers and fathers like a shade being drawn against the sun, the eyes growing wide, the mouths going slack. It is the same expression you sometimes see captured in newspaper photographs of the dispossessed taken in war-torn countries, a haunting, luminescent halo of unutterable sadness and loss, an expression that makes you shiver and look away and thank God that you are not experiencing the emotions caught in that picture. It is what despair looks like, despair that no one but another who has borne it can fully comprehend. Neonatology has come a long way in the last decade, and that look, once all too common, is not often seen in the NICU these days. But it has not been banished, and it is here today, on Susan Bernard's face, as Jose Perez tries to comfort her with quiet words and a fatherly hug.

These are not the moments he envisioned at age thirteen, when he first realized he wanted to be a doctor, this comforting instead of saving, helping children and parents say good-bye. He remembers, then, something he once heard a pastor on the car radio say many years ago, and he repeats it for Susan as he has for other patients who have worn the expression that now settles onto her face.

"Look at it this way," he says quietly, his eyes locked on hers. "You've had the opportunity to personally meet an angel. Because that's his next stop. So you see, you're really very lucky."

He hugs her again. He can feel her tears on his shoulder and, after a few seconds, the motion of her head slowly nodding.

Life in the NICU would be unbearably sad but for one thing: Every day, two or three or four or more babies go home.

This simple fact can be all too easy to forget at times, given the penchant of the Miller Children's NICU for drawing the smallest and sickest babies born all over the region. Such infants absorb the lion's share of time, attention and angst in the neonatal unit, though they represent a minority of the overall patient population. The majority of babies have relatively brief and benign stays in the NICU, and the percentage of infants who survive and are sent home reflects this: More than 97 percent of the babies make it here; that is among the best survival rate in the nation for NICUs that treat the highest-risk patients. The survival rate for the extremely low-birth-weight micropreemies is even more striking—81 percent survive here, compared to a national rate of 65 percent (based on 1997 statistics).

Some of the babies nearing discharge today started out as sick as the babies in Room 288. Some are even sicker. But after three or four months—or three or four days, for the lucky ones, and somewhere in between for the majority—the ventilators are rolled away, the IVs are disconnected, the look of desperation on the parents' faces is replaced by nervous anticipation. Their babies are hearty now, they are greedily sucking up milk, they are losing their preemie thinness and starting to look like the babies in the newborn nursery. They can sit in car seats and not turn blue. They wear regular-sized diapers. They fuss when they're agitated, instead of just losing consciousness and forgetting to breathe. They have survived their hundreds of thousands of dollars' worth of cutting-edge care and, in varying degrees, have begun to thrive.

There is no mistaking the parents in the unit whose children are about to go home: They are carrying huge bundles of goodies and thick packets of instructions assembled by the nurses, and wearing expressions that mirror those on the new parents standing outside that window where the healthy newborns lie. Most of the children require little additional care at home; only about 20 percent of all preemies have some sort of lasting disability or developmental delay, and many of those are minor. (The outlook for the tiniest preemies is less encouraging.) Some of the parents are wheeling oxygen bottles behind them, with respiration monitors slung over their shoulder—safeguards for babies whose lungs are still weak or who still hesitate in their breathing while asleep. Others have bagfuls of medication. Most get a new antiviral drug called Synagis to reduce the likelihood of serious respiratory infections, a far more frequent—and dangerous—problem for former preemies than full-term kids. It doesn't matter, though—it's the going home that they focus on, the healing that is nearing completion.

"This is the best day of my life," one mother gushes as she puts down the car seat with her young son in it so she can hug a favorite nurse good-bye. "I'll never forget you," she whispers. "You saved my baby."

The nurse looks lovingly at the napping infant. He has been transformed from a sickly preemie with gastroschisis, almost as bad as Nikkol Hawkshaw, into an active, happy boy who is well on his way to catching up with nature. He is bright and alert and adorable; even when he was sick and in pain, he looked up at those caring for him with extraordinarily wise, dark eyes that seemed to understand far more than they should. He had been here many months, was transferred to another hospital for successful eye surgery, then came back to finish his recovery. He has come a long, long way—and so has his mother. The terror and helplessness with which she entered the unit have been replaced with firm resolve and the ability to provide the special care her child will need at home—to change his dressings, monitor his vitals, mix his complex formula—as well as any nurse in the unit. They both will be missed.

"We loved having your son here," the nurse says as mother and child go down the hallway toward the elevator, toward the sunshine and a new life. "Almost as much as we love seeing him go."

• • •

Fifty yards away, through two sets of doors, under the bright lights of the OR, Lupe Padilla is waiting for Baby Girl Berger to choose between living and dying.

The only sound in the room comes from a nurse stowing the disposable epinephrine syringe the doctor just injected into the baby. The syringe comes with a peel-off laser-scan tag, just one more item to be counted and tallied on the forms that accompany every piece of equipment in the hospital, even the crash carts, because whether the patient lives or dies, hospital billing is forever.

"Come on, baby," Lupe says again.

Lupe has her crisis look on. Her chapped lips are pursed like a wine taster's, her forehead is a field of furrows. Her face is both serious and expectant, a poker face that betrays nothing but intense interest. This is a good look for a doctor to have, especially when things are going to hell. It connotes gravity without panic. Only those closest to Lupe know just how bad things have to be for this look to appear.

Lupe inherited the look from her father, a self-made man with a tendency to scatter the unusual in his wake. An accountant by trade, Jose Luis Padilla is also a self-taught architect and a quirkily talented homebuilder who doubled the size of his own home over the course of three years' worth of weekends, adding one bedroom after another to accommodate the growing Padilla family—eight children, an assortment of pets, enormous holiday feasts. Then he built a house for one son and renovated another for one of Lupe's sisters. ("Okay," Lupe says, "so the toilet has hot water in one of the houses, and in the other, the electrical system is haunted—you never know which light will come on when you flip a switch. But we like to say that adds to the charm.")

One day, at age sixty-eight, the elder Padilla appeared without warning at Lupe's house in Long Beach and announced, "I need to put on a new roof." He was wearing his own crisis face, and Lupe knew better than to argue. To him, the roof *was* a crisis. When she left for work, he was happily clambering up a ladder.

A few hours later, a call came in to the NICU from Lupe's eleven-

year-old daughter: "Papi fell off the roof." She met her dad in the ER—
he had a compression fracture of the spine, serious though not perma-
nently damaging. His doctor warned Papi to stay off the roof for at least
two weeks. Two weeks and one day later, he was back up there. Prior to
that, he had been on the ladder at the edge of the roof, directing the
work. "I'm not *on* the roof. The doctor said not to go *on* the roof, and so
I stop here!" he shouted down at his daughter when she tried to get him
to rest. Lupe shakes her head whenever she recalls the story: That's why
he wanted her to be a lawyer. They both tend to think this way, looking
for loopholes—he, to elude the toll of years; she, to cheat death one
more time for her patients. Lupe is very much her father's daughter.

Now, in OR-9, she is watching and waiting for Baby Girl Berger to
live or die. How far this code will continue is strictly up to Lupe now,
doctor in the uneasy role of God. When it is known ahead of time that
a baby is in trouble, when tests have shown a birth defect so bad that a
life worth living is just about impossible, the neonatologists meet with
the expectant parents and have terrible discussions: How much in the
way of heroic measures should we do? When should we stop trying to
revive your child? Should we try at all? Even then, with sufficient time
and knowledge to consider the options and probabilities, the parents
find it hard to absorb, harder still to say anything other than, "Do
everything you can to save my baby." Even when there is no hope, they
pray that the predictions were wrong, that a well baby will magically
appear. Lupe hates cases like that; all the neonatologists do. But in this
code, a crisis so out of the blue, so impossible to predict, there was no
reason for any such discussions with the parents. Lupe must rely on her
own knowledge and instinct to do everything possible to save this girl's
life without going too far. But where, she wonders, do you draw the
line? Here? In another minute? Or have I already crossed it?

"Come on, baby," Lupe urges one more time, and a moment later
the infant's mouth opens slightly.

Everyone leans forward a little, as if they aren't quite sure of what
they saw. It is just past the twelve-minute mark. Twelve minutes with-

out breath or heartbeat. The mouth opens a little more, and Baby Girl Berger's chest appears to shake. Then, with a shuddering gasp, she begins to breathe. The last dose of epinephrine at the last possible moment did the trick.

"I've got a pulse," Martha Rivera calls out. Lupe listens to the faltering heart with her stethoscope and watches Martha silently signal the pulse rate by raising and lowering her index finger in time with the beat, the silent, efficient communication of a neonatal Code Blue. The pulse rate starts at forty, then rises to eighty. In less than a minute, she's over a hundred and holding. The code is over, as abruptly as it began.

"Let's get her in a warming blanket and over to the unit," Lupe says. "She's ice cold."

With Greg Moses still bagging the child, Martha lifts the baby, IV lines trailing, into the transport incubator. In a moment, the infant is wheeled from the room, the respiratory therapist jogging alongside, continuing to supply oxygen.

There is a plethora of tests to do, but Lupe feels the likely cause is pulmonary hypertension, a serious ailment in newborns that causes high blood pressure in the arteries leading to the lungs. When the pressure gets high enough, the vessels constrict tightly and blood is shunted away from the lungs, depriving the body of oxygen. It can be caused by the sort of pulmonary hemorrhage Baby Girl Berger experienced at birth, one of the worst traumas a newborn can suffer, and one of the hardest to treat. Hearts, livers, stomachs, intestines and most of the vital organs can be surgically repaired, more or less. Not lungs. Whatever you come into the world with has to keep you alive. The lungs can be assisted, they can be given a chance to heal, but they cannot be fixed the way a surgeon can untwist a bowel or repair an aorta.

The baby is taken to the unit's small treatment room, crammed with equipment, a digital scale and a miniature operating table with lights and a warmer that instantly turns the area around the baby into a sauna. Wearing scrubs, masks and surgical hats is nearly unbearable.

Baby Girl Berger is weighed, measured and given a second umbilical line. The she is placed on a high-frequency oscillating ventilator, which looks like a blue-and-beige box crammed with electronics sitting atop a pedestal on wheels. This is one of the newer and more expensive pieces of equipment in the NICU; it is radically different from the conventional ventilators that force air into and out of a baby's lungs in a rhythm that at least resembles normal respiration. In contrast, the oscillator delivers and sucks out tiny puffs of oxygen hundreds of times a minute rather than whole lungfuls of air. The lungs are not emptied and filled with each breath, but their contents are continually recycled through this oscillation of the air inside. It is thought that the tiny bursts of oxygen cause less trauma to the lungs, although there is still debate among neonatologists as to the value of this machine and how—or even why—it works. The physics of breathing, such as it is understood (and surprisingly, it is understood far less than the physics of space flight or computer chips or quantum particles), suggests that this ventilator shouldn't help at all, but it often does. Lupe needs this device to give the baby's lungs a chance to heal. The force of the high-pressure oxygen should act as a kind of gaseous tourniquet to slow, perhaps stop, the deadly bleeding inside the girl's lungs. A conventional vent at pressures high enough to accomplish this could blow the baby's lungs apart, but the oscillator allows these high settings to be used more safely.

When the lines are in and the oscillator is chugging away, Baby Girl Berger is wheeled into Room 288 and parked in Position Four. After a bit, Harry Berger tentatively walks into the unit, looking at his daughter uncertainly. He is in shock. One minute he was standing in the delivery, excited, suspecting nothing. Now he is in this terrifying place, trying to make sense of what he is seeing. They haven't even chosen a name yet; the tag on the incubator simply reads, "BG Berger." His new baby looks so remote, so far away from him, hidden behind the technology, the hoses, the fear. The oscillator is hardest of all to get used to: His baby does not appear to be breathing. Rather, she vibrates from the action of the machine, her chest and the rest of her body thrumming like a drum skin.

Lupe takes Mr. Berger into the coordinator's office and explains what has been done, the tests they will need to run, how they can do little more for the moment other than wait and see what happens next. She knows this is not the conversation any parents ever imagined when they first learned they would be having a baby. All they expected to hear was girl or boy, pounds and ounces, blues eyes or brown. She watches him try to take it all in as she tells him it is likely that Baby Girl Berger's brain was affected by the long minutes without a heartbeat. Seizures in the next twelve hours are likely, and she will need high doses of phenobarbital to control them. Other symptoms of brain trauma may become apparent in days to come; some may not appear for months or even years.

When they emerge from the office, Lupe is still talking about epi and bicarb and albumen, but Mr. Berger appears incapable of absorbing any more. His eyes are fixed on the terrible vibrations shaking his daughter's entire body even as they keep her alive. Lupe has told him, as gently as she could, that the baby's life has been saved but that her prognosis is up in the air. She might recover completely. She might have suffered irreparable damage. She might fall somewhere between those extremes. They just don't know. Right now, the main concern is dealing with the lung bleeding, which in itself is a major challenge that may require transferring her to another hospital. She may need an experimental treatment with nitric oxide gas that can cure persistent pulmonary hypertension and give her body the oxygen it needs.

"Her lungs are the priority for now," Lupe says. "We can worry about longer-term problems later."

Afterward, in a moment of reflection away from patients and parents, Lupe sounds particularly gloomy, even for her. The adrenaline high of the code has passed, and she looks tired—with a full night on call still ahead of her. She tries to remember if she took her own heart medication, takes her own pulse, decides that she must have swallowed the requisite pill, then mulls over Baby Girl Berger's future.

"There's no way to predict her long-term outlook," she says. "Twelve minutes without a heartbeat is a very long time, though. If I were a betting woman, I'd have to say the prospects are not good."

Then she brightens a bit. "Of course, I'm the unit pessimist, everyone knows that. This way, I get to be pleasantly surprised instead of disappointed. And if there's one thing I've learned here, it's that you just never can tell."

7

Baby Boy Allman is spread out beneath brilliant warming lights as Dr. Pure Tumbaga threads a clear plastic line into one of her patient's umbilical arteries.

The intensity of the heat makes Pure uncomfortable in her heavy surgical garb and mask, but she ignores her discomfort, absorbed in the subtleties of her task. The plastic tube slowly disappears inside the baby, a surprisingly large quantity of it for such a small child, as the neonatal fellow threads this very thin pipeline through the baby's circulatory system until its tip is lodged just outside the heart. The umbilical lines are the best method of getting drugs into and blood out of a baby, because they can be introduced without puncturing the skin, putting nature's own pipeline to good use.

Dr. Tumbaga would have liked to have put a second line into the umbilical vein, which usually is easier to work with than the two tiny arteries, but there was too much damage at delivery, leaving only one good artery. Sometimes the umbilicus gets twisted or crushed, as happened with this child, or the cutting of the cord leaves too little to work with. The procedure is a threading of the needle done in the blind, by touch rather than eyesight, since the tip of the IV line is invisible inside the child. It is a precise procedure, surgery without cutting, and astounding to watch—unless you happen to be related to the child. Imagine putting a lost drawstring back into a pair of sweatpants—but reduce the size by an order of twenty and make the repository of the drawstring as delicate as parchment, as contorted as a mountain road, and filled with blind alleys and wrong turns. Push the wrong way, a venous line ends up in the liver. Push too hard, an arterial line pokes through the delicate lining of an infant blood vessel. It is a painstaking process that Pure mastered long ago on her nearly complete road to becoming an attending physician.

She removes her surgical gloves as a nurse clears away the blue papers and cloth that draped the baby and formed a sterile field. The umbilical line is a lifesaver, but it is also a potential speedway into the body for infections. Sterile surgical procedures at least slow the advance, though nothing can stop it entirely. Sooner or later, the odds are good that a baby with a line left in place long enough will get infected, yet another of the NICU's quicksand trade-offs. Getting lines out is another of the big milestones for a child in the unit, second only to getting off the vent and starting feeds. When the lines are removed, the infection rate drops through the floor: Intact, healthy skin and a vigorous hand-washing policy are the best safeguards against infection yet known to man.

Once the surgical drapes are gone and Baby Boy Allman is uncovered, his shock of blond hair, just like his father's, is in startling contrast to the dark Asian eyes he inherited from his mother. Pure reaches out and touches him gently, her long fingers resting on his chest, as if consoling the unconscious child. It is a gesture she makes almost without thinking. One of the nurses catches the gesture and smiles: Pure touches her patients often, not only because she is a firm believer in the hands-on physical exam, the art of using the feel, sound and appearance of a baby as a critical first diagnostic tool, but because the contact simply seems natural to her, a way of keeping her patients real so they do not become a mere collection of symptoms and syndromes to treat.

This is one of the most valuable lessons Pure has picked up as she nears the end of her training as a neonatal fellow, every bit as important as the skills and science she has absorbed. Some day, she will take her training back with her to her native Philippines, where she hopes to open her own clinic, perhaps an entire hospital. But for now she is content to apply her training here, one baby at a time. Third-year fellows like Pure are one rung below the attending physicians in the medical pecking order. They are certified pediatricians who have signed on for the three more years of NICU clinical work and laboratory research needed to become credentialed specialists in neonatology. They are here to perfect their skills, and, by the time they reach Pure's stage, they can be as good as the attendings. The neonatal fellows operate fairly autonomously, and the third-years, like Pure, have begun to develop their own treatment philosophies. Every neonatologist needs a philosophy, she says, because unlike most other branches of medicine, there is never just one or two accepted ways to treat a preemie—there are dozens. An overarching philosophy is needed to maintain some kind of continuity. If surgeons are the medical world's fearless and precise engineers with their credo being *a chance to cut is a chance to cure,* neonatologists are medicine's artists, relying as much on their own creativity and instinct as they do on exact science in order to deal with the innate unpredictability of preemies.

Now Pure steps away from the new baby and quickly enters medical orders with a light pen on the unit computer behind the incubator: drugs to combat the child's dangerously low blood pressure, antibiotics to ward off infection, surfactant therapy to ease his respiratory distress so he can more quickly wean from the conventional mechanical ventilator hissing and clicking beside him. With the orders complete, Pure double-checks one more time before clicking on enter, absently rubbing her neck with her free hand. The computers in the unit are all positioned at exactly the right height and angle to be ergonomically incorrect, and the doctors all suffer from chronic stiff necks and sore wrists. Yes, Pure sees, the baby's weight and dosage calculations check out and the wristband matches the patient's birth date and name in the computer file:

```
DOB: November 15, 1998
Date of Admission:  November 15, 1998
Name:  Baby Boy Allman
```

Then the neonatal fellow signs off the computer and nods at Art Strauss. The medical director sighs and says, "Finally! Let's get started." The ritual of Morning Rounds at last can begin.

The resident, Valerie Josephson, on her last NICU rotation before becoming a pediatrician, slowly walks over to join Art and Pure so they can begin the traditional counterclockwise rotation around the room, presenting each patient one at a time, reviewing their cases and treatment, with Art peppering the resident and fellow with questions. Part patient care, part learning opportunity, part bull session, Morning Rounds are a mobile classroom in teaching hospitals like Long Beach Memorial. But here, nothing is academic.

Pure presents the first baby, one of the Lee boys. Then it's Valerie's turn. She is lagging behind the other doctors, dragging herself around like a zombie. This in itself is not an unusual sight: Pediatric residents like Valerie—the workhorse occupants of the bottom rung of the medical ladder, doing the routine and the rote for the attendings and being informally trained by the nurses—do three months in the NICU spread over three years. It's not nearly enough time to master its intricacies, so the residents are constantly playing catch-up. They are heavily supervised, heavily worked, barely paid and regularly sleep-deprived. Some residents revel in this chaotic exhaustion; others live in a state of constant dread; most find a measure of both as they catnap between crises in glorified closets called "Call Rooms" just down the hall from the unit, where they forget what their wives and children and boyfriends look like in the crush of sleepless nights away from home. Intubating a crashing two-pound preemie at three in the morning on twenty minutes' worth of sleep is not for the squeamish or the unconfident, which is why many perfectly competent pediatric residents who thought they might want to become neonatologists decide not to sign up for another three years of training after they get a good taste of the NICU. Count Valerie Josephson among this group. Today she looks as if she has had more than enough NICU to last a lifetime, paler than usual beneath her mane of wavy black hair, deep circles rimming her eyes after a long night on call. Residents spend every third night at the hospital, and last night was busy and tough.

Art and Pure look at the resident expectantly, waiting for her to present the twenty-seven-weeker they are standing before, an unstable baby with a possible intraventricular hemorrhage—a brain bleed. The resident opens her file, closes it, opens her mouth to speak, then falters. She winces, rubbing her forehead.

"Rough night?" Art asks with a shaggy raised eyebrow. Valerie offers a weary nod, then suddenly totters, turns white, mutters, "Excuse me," and rushes from the room, about to faint or throw up or both. Art and Pure watch her flee; the medical director deadpans, "Was it something I said?"

Low blood sugar, probably, the resident would later explain: She hadn't eaten since dinner last night. Art shook his head at this. She broke the medical resident's cardinal rule: If you have five minutes, eat; if you have ten, sleep; if you have fifteen, it's a vacation.

Art checks the clock. The list of meetings on his schedule today is like a lead weight in his shirt pocket. And besides the bureaucratic duties, there are more patients to see, an offended parent to placate, a task force to organize, a drug mom to report to a social services agency that will almost certainly do nothing, an insurance crisis to grapple with, a corporate raider angling to steal the entire practice—no one ever said life in the NICU was dull.

He picks up another chart and complains, "I'm never going to get out of here," but the truth is, he doesn't mind very much. Art Strauss will take being in this room over a meeting with hospital bureaucrats any day.

8

BACK IN THE WOMEN'S HOSPITAL, AMALIA ALLMAN IS BEING SUTURED. She is in pain after the difficult labor, but all she can think about is seeing her baby, chafing against the fact that she will not be able to leave the room for several hours. Later, a nurse tells her, they'll take her down to the NICU in a wheelchair. She tries to be patient, but Amalia has a terrible urge to chase after Robert, to see her son, to make sure he's still all right.

Dr. Josefina "Penny" Jacinto, who attended Baby Boy Allman's delivery, has lingered to brief Amalia on the tests and drugs to be administered to her son. The neonatologist assures her that the baby looks stable and, given his stage of development and relatively large size as preemies go, that he should do fine.

"He really looks pretty big," Penny says, betraying the neonatologist's unusual point of view (full-term babies look enormous to these doctors so used to micropreemies). "And he really looked like he turned toward your husband's voice when he said hello."

They both laugh at this. After the baby was finally extracted after many failed attempts and he was handed over to the neonatal team at the warming table, Robert had stood near his son's head and leaned over. In the same exaggerated voice he had used for months when addressing the round bulge of Amalia's stomach, he had called, "Helloooooo, Elias!" They had decided on his name long before, and the word "hello" was stretched out the way a person might call into a mountain crevasse, hoping to find an echo. It had become Robert's nightly ritual. The nurse, the respiratory therapist and Dr. Jacinto had all laughed when they heard this odd call, but they swore to Amalia that the baby seemed to turn his head toward the familiar greeting. Robert had been so excited, saying, "He knows my voice!"

"I just think it's a very good omen," Penny says.

Amalia nods. She likes this petite, perfectly coiffed physician, feels comforted by the fact that every one of her hairs is in place, her nails are beautiful, her clothes appear as immaculate as if they had just come off a hanger. Dr. Jacinto seems to exude professionalism and competence. As a former employee of Nordstrom, the West's most upscale department store, Amalia appreciates Penny's gift for maintaining an unruffled appearance under even the most trying of circumstances. Things must not be so bad if her baby's doctor can look so good, Amalia figures.

The NICU, it seems, is staffed by happy opposites. Penny is in every way the converse of Lupe's pleasantly rumpled disorganization. She only recently gave in to peer pressure and started wearing trousers and loafers instead of skirts and heels at work—but only when she's on overnight call. And even then, at three in the morning, when paged for an emergency, Penny appears in an instant with her hair—and her teeth—freshly brushed. No one has yet figured out how she does it. While the other doctors struggle all day to complete their work following a night on call, Penny somehow always seems to manage to wrap up early and leave on time, every one of her patients dealt with, her charts up to date. She is possessed of a near-photographic memory for names and birth dates and even parents' names, some from more than a decade ago. None of the other neonatologists can remember all the patients' names from one day to the next, much less year to year—there are just too many of them. They can all recite the purely medical information: diagnoses, treatments, outcomes. But Penny remembers the birthdays of kids she treated in 1984.

Penny has a knack for efficiently explaining the complex medical issues to parents, neither confusing nor condescending, and Amalia appreciates this as much as she did Dr. Jacinto's calm efficiency in the delivery room. The first priority, the doctor explains, will be treating the baby's respiratory distress—he'll get help from a ventilator, and possibly from a drug called surfactant to promote lung maturity. Because of his severe bruising, he'll also get phototherapy, to keep the blood waste-product bilirubin from building up in his body, the cause of jaundice. He will get an ultrasound of his vital organs, an X ray of his chest and an echocardiogram of his heart. His blood will be tested for infections and for its chemistry. He will be kept NPO for now—a Latin acronym for "nothing by mouth"—with his nutrition provided intravenously. That could change quickly, and Penny reminds Amalia that she will need to start pumping breast milk, which will be stored in a freezer in the unit, then fed to Elias through a tube placed down his throat. Many weeks will pass before he is capable of sucking and swallowing his nourishment, but that too will come, the neonatologist assures her. She should be prepared for both progress and occasional setbacks, because Elias will be in the unit at least three months, Penny warns.

"I'll see you downstairs later on." Then the doctor leaves the room to return to her patients in the NICU.

Amalia has kept a journal during her ten days in the hospital, entering her daily thoughts as she lay in bed, hoping her premature contractions would stay dormant. Now it will be a journal of Elias's experiences in the NICU, and it is time for the first entry since the delivery. She is writing it in the form of letters to her son, and she has made a conscious decision to be as lighthearted as possible, whether she feels like it or not.

Dearest Elias,

Well, today was your BIRTHDAY! You were born at 11:45 a.m.
this morning. Three pounds, six ounces and fifteen inches long! !
The staff here says you are BIG for twenty-eight weeks. I'm so
glad!! . . . At first I was scared because your whole head was purple!

You got quite bruised on the way out. But after I heard you cry, I

knew you were okay.

She puts the black leather-bound journal aside a moment. What do you say to a baby whose life is so fragile and future so uncertain? she wonders. How do you express the love and hope and fear all tied up in this moment? Should she even try? Will he even want to read this stuff? A darker thought pushes its way into her head then: Will he have a *chance* to read it?

Amalia shakes her head. She will allow no doubts to occupy her thoughts, only the certainty that her child will be fine. She heard him cry, didn't she? Dr. Jacinto sounded so positive, didn't she? He turned his head to his father, didn't he? Everyone laughed at it, a wonderful moment, as if the sun had just peeked out from behind a cloud. That wouldn't have happened if Elias weren't going to be okay, Amalia told herself. God would never be so cruel.

She finishes the entry:

> *Everything went great and Daddy was a great coach! ! He was*
>
> *helping me count during the pushing and was by my side the entire*
>
> *time. . . . We both love you so much and want you to grow and get*
>
> *healthy.*
>
> *Love, Mommy*

She looks at all the blank pages in the thick journal, which is supposed to begin and end with Elias's days in the NICU, and she has a sudden pang of fear: The last thing she wants is to have enough to write about to fill the entire book.

9

LISA LEE IS A FIGHTER, HAS BEEN ALL HER LIFE. IT IS LITTLE WONDER, then, that her three babies are fighters as well.

"They are very, very strong," she says with pride whenever someone asks how her children are doing. Not better or worse, not sick or well. *Strong.* She says the word in her lilting accent almost as if it were an incantation. It is an odd thing to say about immobilized preemies hooked up to innumerable IVs and mechanical ventilators, but she has a point: These kids have made it through more than most people endure in a lifetime. Their continued survival defies the odds.

Eric Kuan Te Lee, Marlon Kuan Shin Lee, and Osmond Kuan Hue Lee were born a month ago after little Eric, a tough guy even in the womb, kicked a hole in the fetal membrane (commonly known as the water bag) with a foot the size of a thumbnail. This brought on premature labor at an impossibly early point in the pregnancy: twenty-two weeks. Lisa was given magnesium sulfate to stop contractions (no one is sure why it works or how well it works, but it is one of the few treatments available); betamethasone, a steroid used in a skin cream for adult eczema, was injected into Lisa Lee's bloodstream because it has the additional property of accelerating lung development in preemies; and antibiotics were given to combat the inevitable infections that occur once the barrier of the placenta has been breached. Complete bed rest was prescribed, a difficult pill for her to swallow, because Lisa Lee rarely rests. Somehow, though, she knew she had to keep the babies for another two weeks. She had to make it to the twenty-four-week thresh-old, no matter what, so that her babies would have a fighting chance.

That she might not succeed did not ever occur to her, and if she had any doubts, she would rather choke on the words than utter them aloud. Ever since she grew up in Taiwan in the 1950s, struggling for a place in a world that did not open many doors for young Chinese girls, Lisa Lee has made the endurance of hardships, the assumption of bur-dens, and a bedrock stoicism that acknowledges no pain a virtual reli-gion. When she and her family visit the babies, the others shed tears or lose control. Not Lisa Lee. It is the mother of these sick children who comforts the others. No matter that she herself is sick, that she is bleed-ing internally and needs transfusions, possibly a hysterectomy. She dis-misses inquiries from the nurses about her health with a nod and a smile. "I'm fine," she always says. "What about the boys?"

Her steely resolve seems to have begun by the time she was five. Her older sister, crippled by polio and forced to wear braces, was mocked by other children, an easy target of cruelty. Though two years her junior, Lisa became her sister's protector, walking her to school each day and fighting off the tormentors with fists, kicks and bites. She put off her own schooling to help her sister get through school. Later, she spent years caring for their father when he fell ill from a stroke. She built her own import-export business, supporting her entire family. Eventually she brought her business to America and moved to the suburb of La Verne, east of Los Angeles, though her husband, for all but a handful of days each year, remains in Taiwan.

Her chief desire was to have children of her own, a desire that was frustrated year after year by her health problems: high blood pressure, a bout with hepatitis, and an ectopic pregnancy that ended in miscar-riage. She was diagnosed with infertility five years ago and, at age forty-two, resorted to *in vitro* fertilization and embryo implantation. The ten-thousand-dollar procedure—which is not covered by medical in-surance—worked. But in the process, Lisa Lee became one of the thou-sands of women who found that fertility treatments had brought her several children—damaged children—instead of the one healthy baby she sought.

Beneath their professional detachment, the neonatologists simmer with anger over such pregnancies because they know they are largely avoidable: The best means of treating premature birth, they like to say, is *preventing* premature birth. There are alternative techniques that would reduce the likelihood of high-risk multiple births and the complications that go with them, and many fertility specialists—like those at Long Beach Memorial—use them. But others, operating with little regulation and eyes firmly on the bottom line, shy away from these techniques because they also lower the likelihood of conception on the first try, thus increasing costs. Once pregnant with three or five or seven babies, many families refuse the option of reducing the number of embryos because it is a form of abortion.

Yet statistics paint a stark picture. The advent of unregulated fertility treatments is the main reason why twins are born at a rate 50 percent greater than in 1980. The increase in the rate of triplets and higher numbers of multiples has been even more dramatic in the course of those same twenty years: more than 400 percent.

These days the NICU in Long Beach is almost never without quads or triplets, once a rarity, most of them fertility-treatment babies. The risk that these babies will be premature or sick or both has increased proportionately as well, particularly with older, medically fragile mothers like Lisa Lee. The fact that infant mortality in the United States, particularly among preemies, is greater than in many other developed nations can be linked directly to this epidemic of fertility-induced multiple births. Art Strauss derides this phenomenon as "unregulated human experimentation." The higher-order multiples that sometimes result from the most aggressive fertility treatments—six or more babies at a time—are the most harrowing to a neonatologist. "The human body simple wasn't built to deliver litters," Lupe grumbles when news of the latest "miracle mom" hits the papers—fertility-induced octuplets in Texas, all of them seriously ill.

The members of the NICU staff are as critical of the mass media's handling of this issue as they are of the overly aggressive treatments themselves—a gauzy glamorization of artificially induced multiple births as miracles rather than the unintended medical miscalculations they often can be. This sort of coverage peaked with the birth of the McCaughey septuplets in 1997, when magazines and television shows gushed over the miracle births and the family sustained by unprecedented armies of volunteers and contributors. The problem, from a neonatologist's point of view, is the false impression the public gets from such cases, in which all the babies ultimately recovered and went home—the happy endings making for good press but lousy examples of day-to-day realities in the NICU. They fear that such skewed publicity allays concerns about irresponsible fertility treatments when concerns should in fact be mounting. Indeed, the technique has become so popular that there are now an estimated 150,000 human embryos in medical freezers around the country, awaiting implantation, with more and more couples opting for treatments all the time. These treatments are a blessing for most who seek them out. But lost in the hype is the fact that many multiple, premature births end tragically, without extravagant headlines, volunteer baby-sitters or the word "miracle" being uttered even once. The Lee boys are living proof of this sad equation: their mother had no idea what she was getting into.

Of course, if you ask her now, knowing all the risks and problems, she says she would not change a thing. She has been blessed with three boys. How could she wish any one of them had not been born? "They are a gift to me," she says. "I love them all. I *want* them all."

After her labor was halted by drugs, Lisa was able to hold on for thirteen days of bed rest, bringing the boys to exactly the twenty-four-week threshold needed to at least even the odds for survival. At that point, her obstetrician tried to deliver only Eric, but his attempts failed, and all three babies were born at once. The OR was so crowded with the personnel needed for three very sick triplets that one of the neonatal teams had to wait outside with a transport incubator and work on Osmond in the hall.

All three babies were very sick. Marlon—Baby Boy Two—was in severe septic shock, an infection so intense that his blood was filled with toxins that threatened to overwhelm his organs and immune system before antibiotics could slow down the invasion. Osmond—Baby Boy Three—who possessed the worst lungs, quickly went on the oscillating ventilator and stayed there, his respiration a mess. Eric—ironically, the "troublemaker," as Lisa Lee calls him, again with a tinge of pride, as if it had been moxie at work when he kicked his way into the world—was the healthiest of the bunch. He progressed to Room 276, the less intensive step-down room, in less than three weeks while his brothers' survival was still touch and go. There he "self-extubated"—he literally pulled out his breathing tube. The staff of the NICU likes to see this. They say the baby knows when he's ready, that if he has the strength to free himself from the noxious tube down his throat, then he's probably strong enough to get by without it. And Eric did pretty well for several days without the vent, feeding heartily and gaining weight for the first time from calories rather than retained fluids. But then, with grower-and-feeder status tantalizingly close, a massive infection sent him crashing back to Room 288, where he remains the sickest of the three brothers, his feedings halted, his kidneys showing signs of failing, his doctors unable to find the key to reversing his fragile, wounded body's insistent decline.

His chart overflows its binder, mute testimony to a lifetime worth of medical effort crammed into a month, page after page of tests, treatments and reports, dry and clinical. A grainy Polaroid of Lisa is taped to a cover page, an ID photo so the nurses will recognize her when she comes in at any hour. It was taken the day the boys were born; she wears a hospital gown and a hopeful expression mixed with pain. Opposite this page is the "Birth Souvenir," a certificate just like the families in the newborn nursery get, complete with the baby's footprints in smudged black ink.

But Eric's ghostly footprints, though perfect in their humanity, are impossibly little, the smallest toe no bigger than the head of a pin.

Osmond's chart is just as swollen as his brothers', the general rule being that the thicker the chart, the sicker the baby. His main problem is a heart defect. It is common in preemies, but it must be repaired before it slowly kills him. The surgery is scheduled for today. Lisa Lee came in an hour before the operation was scheduled to begin and prayed next to her son for a long time. Then she began to rub his feet, using the ancient Chinese art of acupressure to try to heal his organs. When she was through, she gave an impromptu massage lesson to some of the nurses.

"Got a headache?" she asks. "Just rub your big toe hard. It works, really."

"How do you stay so cheerful?" one of the nurses asks her. "I would be a basket case if I were you."

"Well, I stay strong for my boys," she says simply. "I can't let them see me lose control. It wouldn't be good for them." She looks into Osmond's incubator, willing him to open his eyes, which he does on occasion, seemingly to exchange glances with his mother. But today they stay shut, and she sighs. "I have to stay strong for him today. So he will come back to me."

It is no small irony that the starting point for all this, the newly conceived embryo, is a hearty thing, far sturdier than the fetus it will soon become and infinitely more durable than the delicate Lee babies and their fellows in Room 288, clinging to life inside their incubators.

A new embryo has to be tough, for its journey to the womb is rough and difficult, which is why scientists have found it can also be removed, manipulated, stored, frozen and carried around as safely as a pint of ice cream. And ironically, it is these qualities that have made modern fertility treatments—and their complications—possible.

This impervious stage of embryonic development passes all too quickly. Once placed in the uterus (by nature or science), the developing embryo in short order becomes utterly dependent on the mother for survival. For the next six months, it will remain as fragile as a snowflake.

In the first month of gestation, the embryo seems to fold in on itself, forming a variety of tubes and chambers as a vague mass of cells begins to take on a human-tadpole shape. Long before ultrasound and fiber-optic technology brought us images of this remarkable transformation, the ancient Greek philosopher Aristotle correctly described this process and called it epigenesis, the rise of order out of chaos. It took two thousand years for science to discard the rack of bogus, silly and sometimes harmful theories of human development that came after Aristotle and to return to his accurate and elegant theory.

Three weeks after conception, the embryo has a beating heart and the beginnings of a circulatory system, though the tiny organ has not yet fully divided into separate chambers. That will happen by the end of the eighth week, like a flower budding, then closing in on itself, an incredible genesis that, despite its baffling complexity, almost always comes out right. But not every time: If the balletic flowering of tissues and pathways is flawed or incomplete, through the effects of a bad gene, a toxin, a disease or a random mutation, that child will be born with a heart defect. It happens this early, though the malformation may remain undetected right up until birth.

The embryonic heart also comes equipped with an intentional defect called a *patent ductus arteriosus,* which in the second month of gestation begins to divert circulation away from the budding lungs and back to the heart, an eminently sensible arrangement for an embryo, which gets its oxygen from the placenta, not its inert, undeveloped lungs. In full-term newborns, this PDA closes automatically, nature's planned obsolescence. But preemies lack the necessary hormone to shut this extra vessel, and what was an efficient bypass *in utero* becomes a deadly time bomb outside the womb. Out in the real world, the flow through the open PDA reverses at birth, turning the bypass into a floodgate, filling a preemie's lungs with so much fluid they can no longer function properly, a debilitating and ultimately fatal condition if uncorrected. Powerful drugs that act in place of the missing hormone can shut the PDA (at the risk of causing kidney failure), but in very small or very sick babies, surgery on the delicate arteries around the heart may be needed. This is the surgery Osmond Lee is about to undergo, an operation that was set in motion many months before, in the quiet, crowded space of the womb.

At the four-week mark, the healthy embryo is three eighths of an inch long and weighs less than a gram. That's one twenty-eighth of an ounce, less than an aspirin tablet. Yet there are already bulges extending from the front of the brain—the first hint of eyes—and, along the torso, small, smooth buds that will become arms and legs. A month later, the embryo is an inch long and has increased its weight fourfold. All the major organs have begun to form: the liver, the stomach, the kidneys, though the smallest of these crucial, delicate organs are not much bigger than the head of a pin. Until this stage, all embryos are female; now sexual differentiation begins, but only if certain chemicals are released that transform the organism into a male. It is also at this stage that certain rare defects begin to occur: abnormalities in the brain, extra openings or missing openings in the throat or abdomen or spine, intestines that are given a doorway to form outside the body instead of within.

By week twelve, the embryonic stage ends and the fetal stage begins. There are fingers and toes and the placenta is fully formed. The weight of the fetus is now sixty grams—just over two ounces. During the next four weeks, the fetus will be able to suck and make breathing movements. There is hair and the ability to hear. Meconium—fetal feces— start to form in the bowels. Blood vessels begin to form in the retina, a very delicate process that accelerates in the last three months of pregnancy and that can be disrupted by premature birth—which is why premature babies so often have lifelong problems with their eyes.

By twenty weeks, the fetus is eight inches and ten ounces—the size and weight of an average hot dog and bun. The gelatinous skin is covered with fine hair called lanugo, a thin, furry coat that disappears by birth but that is often present on preemies. The whitish protective secretion, *vernix caseosa,* will form a few weeks later to cover the delicate skin in pasty layers, almost as if it were troweled on. Perhaps it is nature's way of compensating for the absence of fat under the skin—subcutaneous fat does not begin to form until the thirtieth week of gestation, which is why most preemies look like wrinkled, skinny old men. And it is why they cannot control their own temperature and why fluid evaporates from inside their bodies in a dehydrating rush, like dew boiling off the grass at sunrise. There's no insulation to keep it in.

By the twenty-fourth week, at the end of the sixth month of pregnancy, a healthy fetus weighs somewhere between a pound and a pound and a half and can be as long as twelve inches. The nervous system is functioning and hypersensitive, easily overwhelmed by too much stimulation, which is why a parent's gentle stroke can seem painful to a micropreemie. The visual and auditory centers of the brain are not fully developed as yet, although taste and smell, our most primitive mammalian senses, are far more intense and attuned than they will ever be again. An infant, even a preemie, can differentiate his mother's milk by smell and taste from a hundred others'.

Fifteen years ago, babies born at this stage were called miscarriages. Even ten years ago, survival was very much in question. Today, more often than not, they survive with aggressive use of drugs, mechanical ventilation and emergency resuscitation, just as the Lee triplets in Room 288 were brought back from the brink. Many babies born at this stage today will not only survive, they will thrive, with few or no lasting aftereffects. But there is no guarantee that a life saved will be a life worth living. The million-dollar miracle that is a twenty-four-weeker does not necessarily come neatly equipped with a happy ending: pain, loss and disability burden some of those who survive such early admission to the world. As many as half of these micropreemies will have visual impairment because of blood-vessel abnormalities in their retinas; most will do fine with glasses, but some will be much worse, and a few will be blind. Many will have at least some developmental delays; a significant number face cerebral palsy and lung disease.

The road to wellness for these babies is a difficult one. They come into the world with organs that are fully formed but not necessarily fully functional. The complex brain chemistry of the central nervous system that instigates the urge to breathe, and the simple coordination needed to suck and swallow without choking to death, are not yet in place. The blood vessels in the twenty-four-weeker's brain are extremely delicate and prone to intraventricular hemorrhage—they burst and bleed, sometimes leaving devastating swaths of damage, hydrocephalus, and a need for multiple brain surgeries. Their immune systems barely work, and infections as simple as a cold virus can kill. Their stomachs and intestines are not ready to digest food, leaving them subject to clogging, inflammation and infection—a deadly condition with an ugly name, Necrotizing Enterocolitis, drawn from the ancient Greek word for death, *nekros*. The name is literal: When a baby gets NEC, the bowels literally begin to die inside the child's gut. The diseased portions of the bowel—sometimes most of it—must be cut out, and what's left must be mended like scraps, a process called resection.

The Lee triplets have, to varying degrees, suffered from all of these things, and more. The worst, though, is the problem of their lungs: Twenty-four-weekers simply lack the strength to breathe fast enough and deep enough to stay alive. Even intubation and mechanical ventilators provide only a short-term fix, for the smallest preemie lungs lack a critical substance, surfactant, a natural Teflon that maintains surface tension inside the delicate fabric of the lungs. Surfactant safeguards the lung's tiny air sacs, which fill and empty with each breath and transfer oxygen to the blood vessels webbing the fabric of the lungs. Without surfactant, the sacs begin adhering, scarring and closing down. The oxygen is there, but it can't get to the bloodstream. Higher and higher pressures on the ventilator have to be used to compensate for the damage, to keep the baby from asphyxiating. That causes more damage still, and getting them off the machine then becomes like climbing a mountain. In twenty-four-weekers, surfactant must be provided artificially; twenty-eight-weekers have a bit of their own but usually not enough. Thirty-two- to thirty-four-weekers without complications are golden: Usually, though not in every case, they can breathe on their own.

It is along this continuum that medicine begins its uneasy dance with law and ethics, morality and the politics of abortion and choice. Somewhere between the twenty-second and twenty-eighth week of gestation, running along the border of the second and third trimesters of pregnancy, the fetus becomes "viable." It is a cold word, a clinical word that means different things to different ears, and the definition seems to change not only with the year's scientific developments but with the setting in which the question is posed: church or courtroom, boardroom or ballot box, the answer is fluid. But in practical terms, in the language of the NICU (as well as in Supreme Court rulings), viability starts with a full six months in the womb. After that, most premature babies without other life-threatening conditions can survive. Before that, most will die. There is some debate over whether this line is best anchored in the twenty-third week or the twenty-fourth, and it varies hospital to hospital, region to region, country to country (the United States, for instance, routinely goes all out with infants that are to this day considered miscarriages in other parts of the world). This line shifts for babies with birth defects, organ failure, genetic disorders and overwhelming infections that can tip the scales against viability right up to a full-term pregnancy. The twenty-four-week line applies only when everything else goes *right*. The problem is, premature birth is often brought on because something else has gone wrong with the baby, the mother or both. It's almost always a double whammy, which is why drawing firm lines in the NICU can be maddeningly difficult.

For all of medicine's awesome accomplishments, the engineering that makes a child viable, that governs the transformation of egg into person, dwarfs anything constructed by human ingenuity—no computer chip, concrete-and-glass tower or Egyptian pyramid could begin to compare. No one but nature could construct a human brain, a tiny lump of convolutions and connections that, if built in a linear fashion by the human hand, would have to be ten feet long in order to provide the storage capacity inside an infant's head. No human could build anything that begins to work like the placenta, nature's perfect isolation tank, vault and bunker rolled into one, an organ that arises out of nothingness to afford a level of protection for the fetus that no human will ever experience again. The placenta—from the Latin word for "circular cake" and thought by the ancients to be the receptacle of the soul—shields the fetus from disease and from the mother's own immune system (which would otherwise attempt to destroy the embryo like an invading parasite) while also drawing nutrition, oxygen and other vital elements from the mother's bloodstream without ever actually touching the mother's blood. The placenta's miraculous properties allow even mothers with AIDS to bear children who are free of the HIV virus. Even the baby's skull is a masterpiece of tectonic engineering, built of bony plates that can stretch and move and assume a conical shape during the crushing forces of delivery, spreading the pressures of birth over the entire surface of the skull to spare the precious brain from injury, then allow it to grow at an astonishing rate.

What the neonatologist knows is that even the best engineering sometimes fails. The slightest misstep along the way, in the formation of the heart or the plates of the skull or the closure of the palate or the structure of the abdominal wall, and the baby becomes an NICU patient. And then the only questions that matter to a neonatologist are: Is this new life viable? Can this tiny organism sustain itself outside the womb?

In the NICU, the vexing question of when life begins, which has sparked so much anger and debate, pales next to the far more practical question of when survival can be imagined. Or should be.

For Baby Boy Lee Three, his heart surgery may well provide the answer.

. . .

"Do you know the tensile strength of the descending aorta of a twenty-four-weeker?" the surgeon asks one of the NICU residents, Jason Clark, a bald and jovial second-year whose wife had a baby just two nights ago. A resident's life being what it is, Jason is already on call in the unit tonight. He shakes his head.

Dr. Humberto Ravelo, the cardiothoracic surgeon preparing to operate on one of the Lee triplets' hearts, beckons for Jason to follow him from the infant's incubator to one of the hand-washing sinks against the wall in Room 288. Ravelo yanks a towel from the wall dispenser, soaks it under the tap, then grasps it between both hands, as if he were about to do a television endorsement for the absorbency of paper cleaning products. He thrusts the sopping towel at Jason and says, "Just like this."

Then he pulls ever so gently. The towel shreds limply into sodden tatters. "That's what it's like with these little guys," he says. "The arteries are wet paper. One false move, and it's all over. One little tear, and their chest fills with blood. They bleed out before you can do a thing."

Jason shakes his head, impressed, as Ravelo intended, a typical surgeon in this regard: capable of doing the incredible and unashamed about pointing it out. He is the only surgeon in the medical center who routinely does the PDA operations in preemies. No one else wants to touch them. Ravelo throws away the pieces of towel and returns to the baby, clucking like a disgruntled hen at his latest lab results while the nurse preps the baby for surgery.

"This kid's a fighter," Donna assures Ravelo, as she refastens a blue, handmade name tag to the incubator. The nurses make them for all their patients; this one has the baby's official hospital designation, Lee—BBTHREE, followed by a heart, surrounding the baby's first name in gentler script, Osmond. A lock of wispy brown hair is taped to the tag, baby's first haircut. "He's had all kinds of death dives," Donna tells the surgeon, "when we think we're going to lose him. But he's just one of those babies who wants to live."

The surgery takes place in the NICU's treatment room, the glorified storage closet. One door opens into Room 288, the other leads to the hallway to the ORs, where C-sections are performed. The treatment room is where babies are brought when they need to be worked on before entering the NICU. It is also where various medical supplies are stored on shelves in the back—the space-hungry unit has to use whatever it's got. And, when necessary, the treatment room becomes an operating theater—once again, bringing the hospital to the baby, instead of vice versa.

Present are two surgical nurses, an anesthesiologist, a surgeon to assist, and Dr. Ravelo who, by extraordinary coincidence, is another Cuban-American child of the Pedro Pan smuggling operation, working side by side with Jose Perez.

Osmond Lee lies on a treatment table under the intense radiance of a heat lamp, hoses and IV lines leading from him to the anesthesiologist's machinery. He looks very much like a miniature old man, prone, wizened and bruised-looking, skin the color and texture of an overripe peach. His eyes are puffy and tightly shut. The only motion visible is the slight rise and fall of his sparrow chest, kept in motion by the square beige box of the ventilator puffing next to him. The device's implacable computer imager traces the asymmetrical and flattened inhalation pattern of badly damaged lungs, a kind of zigzagging ellipse instead of the healthy oval shape normal infant lungs produce. Unable to feed and dependent on intravenous nourishment, Osmond Lee has gained only a few ounces since his birth weight of 628 grams, which was just an eyelash over one pound, six ounces, one fifth to one sixth a normal newborn's size. Osmond Lee, in other words, entered the world about the size and weight of the average kitten, his smallness intensified by the fact that he had to share space and nourishment with two brothers. His eyes were fused shut, his skin was translucent and covered with fetal down, his blood anemic, his body riddled with infection.

The infection has been tamed for the moment, his blood's lack of red cells and platelets boosted by some fifty transfusions in less than a

month. But now his PDA must be dealt with. Everything from Osmond's lung function to his ability to eat to his immune system should
improve if the operation is successful. He could go from being the sickest of the triplets to the healthiest in a matter of days.

The baby is given a sedative for sleep, a narcotic for pain, a numb-
ing agent for the surgical site, all in minute doses. Neonatal anesthesia
is a relatively new development. Until fifteen years ago, before Ravelo
began operating on preemies, prevailing medical wisdom held that the
smaller premature babies had such underdeveloped neural pathways
that they sensed little about the outside world and could not even feel
pain. This belief was so ingrained that surgeries were routinely performed without anesthesia or painkillers, just a paralyzing drug so that
the babies would hold still while the surgeons operated. This belief
about the nervous system of preemies turned out to be utterly false, an
unproven, unscientific assumption transformed into gospel by the
weight of years. Generations of premature babies were inadvertently
abused because of this misconception. Now we know that a premature
baby's ability to sense pain—and to be overwhelmed by it—is even
greater than our own.

"Okay, we're ready," the anesthesiologist says, peeking at the patient, then returning to his monitors, needles and gauges.

The nurses move quickly to wash Osmond and drape him with
sterile blue paper, tucking and taping. In a few minutes, his entire body
is covered except for the incision area along his left side. The skin there
is sterilized with brown Betadine solution.

Ravelo is seated in front of the baby on a tall stool, a light and magnifying binoculars strapped to his head like a pilot's visor. He jokes with
the team that he always used to stand during surgery as a matter of
principal—until he turned fifty last year. "Now I sit. As a matter of
principal." He sits erect, a broad man in dark blue scrubs, his salt-and-
pepper hair close-cropped.

Ravelo peers through the binoculars and makes some adjustments
to the draping, adding some tape, pulling things into place. He draws a

line where the incision will go and then he begins, cutting into the small body with a half-size scalpel, then cauterizing the wound as he goes with a tool called a Bovie. The Bovie looks a great deal like a small soldering iron, tipped by a searing hot needle that seals off blood vessels and minimizes blood loss. The tool produces an uncomfortable sizzle and the rank smell of burning iodine and skin. Ravelo has insisted that there be fifty cubic centimeters of blood on hand for the baby— more than enough to replace Osmond's entire blood supply—but his goal is to wield the Bovie in such a way as to use no blood at all.

His hands move with precision. There is little conversation; the small, hot room is tense with concentration. The image of the tearing paper towel is a powerful one hanging over the proceedings.

"There's really only one word to describe what it's like working on these little ones," the anesthesiologist says midway through the operation. "Scary."

In just a few minutes, the papery skin along Osmond's side has been pulled back, the sheath of muscles over the ribs cut and folded over, and the rib cage parted. The ribs are no bigger than matchsticks. Retractors are used to pry the incision open and the left lung is gently moved aside, revealing two identical pulsing vessels the size of elbow macaroni. The hole in the baby's side is gaping in proportion to his body, but it is still too small to admit Ravelo's fingers or even standard surgical instruments; he has to use small extenders on his tools in order to navigate the tiny jigsaw puzzle inside Baby Boy Lee.

Ravelo's task now is to take some surgical silk and tie off the PDA like the ends of a sausage, a process called ligation. This will shut the PDA, and blood then will be forced through the body instead of overfilling and incapacitating the lungs.

"Okay, there's the culprit," Ravelo says, identifying the PDA. "It's a big one. Let's do it." The nurse hands him the moist silk suture material and his fingers dance, a delicate threading not unlike the motions a fisherman makes when tying flies.

The PDA is a large vein that parallels the descending aorta. The two can look almost exactly alike and thus are prone to being confused. "Of course, if I ligate the wrong one," Ravelo says, "it's game over." Unlike the life-threatening PDA, the aorta is the most essential pipeline sustaining the body. If it were ligated, death would be inevitable, so he checks, double-checks, then checks again the origins and end points of the two vessels, making sure he has correctly identified the PDA before wrapping the surgical silk around it.

There is only one brief scare: In the middle of the surgery, Osmond's heart rate dips suddenly, from a solid 170 beats per minute to 79. Ravelo backs off for a moment. Then the heart rate levels off. Everything is fine.

Twenty-five minutes after the first incision, it is done. The ribs, muscles and skin are stitched together and the wound is glued, bandaged and taped shut. A few minutes later, Osmond is back in his spot in Room 288, and Ravelo is fanning himself with a piece of paper from the chart.

"Remember that television show *Medical Center,* and Dr. Gannon, he did every kind of surgery and he'd always come out with just this perfect little triangle of sweat on his scrubs? Well, this is what happens in the real world." Ravelo looks down at his shirt. It is dark with sweat, soaked through, top to bottom, back and front. He looks as if he just came in from the rain. It is the only sign that he felt any stress during the surgery. He ducks out and quickly pulls on a fresh shirt, then reappears.

"Now let me go talk to the mother," he says, striding into the unit and putting an arm around Lisa Lee, who is beaming at her newly returned son inside the incubator as if he just won the science fair.

"Did it go okay?" she asks eagerly.

"Better," Ravelo responds. "Osmond did great."

"Well, he's strong, you know," Mrs. Lee says with a small smile. "Very strong."

10

Dear Elias,

I should tell you about the first time I saw you . . .

After you were born, they took you directly to the Intensive Care Unit, so I really didn't get to see you. After my recovery, they brought me back to my room. Later that day, Daddy wheeled me over to the unit. Finally.

The first time I saw your face I started to cry . . . they were tears of joy. I was so overwhelmed, I actually have a baby boy!! I fell instantly in love with you. You are an angel sent from heaven.

I pray that you get better soon. I think about you all day and dream about you all night. I love you, Elias.

Love, Mommy

AMID THE NOISE AND HASTE OF ROOM 288, A QUIET WOMAN IN street clothes and a sterile gown reaches unhurriedly into an incubator for one of Art Strauss's patients and gently takes the child from her plastic box. The woman stands out among the other members of the NICU staff in their surgical scrubs and medical gear and hypervigilant postures. She is deliberate and relaxed, though her eyes are watchful.

Sara Masur, the unit's occupational therapist, has arrived to begin working with one of the oldest babies in the NICU.

Art Strauss had asked Sara to consult on the case of five-month-old Nikkol Hawkshaw, for whom the tide never seems to turn. Nikkol has just come off the ventilator after a very long fight to breathe on her own. The child is still on shaky ground, an alarm waiting to happen, and she could slide back into ventilator dependence at any moment. This would shatter the unit's fledgling attempts to get her to eat, and Sara is here to help keep that from happening.

Nikkol is a gastroschisis baby, one of three in the unit recovering from this condition or a similar one called omphalocele. Nikkol's is by far the worst. Her birth defect stems from a failure of the abdominal wall to close during her first few months in the womb. This caused her intestines, liver and a portion of her stomach to form outside her body while she developed *in utero*, where amniotic fluid proved as corrosive as battery acid to the delicate organs. The tubes of bowel, which should have been healthy and pink, were gray and matted at birth, a very bad sign. Complicating matters was the sheer physics of the human body: With nothing taking up space inside her abdomen as it formed, she was born with a tiny wasp waist and precious little room for the organs that belonged there. So when surgeons put the damaged organs back into place, her lungs had to be crowded upward to make room, a literally named process called surgical reduction. Nikkol needed six separate reduction surgeries; the typical case requires only two or three. The crowding of organs has made breathing very, very difficult for her, as if someone were sitting on her chest each time she tries to breathe. The cause of this defect, which occurs in about one in twenty thousand births, is unknown. A higher-than-average incidence in the agricultural regions of Central California, particularly among Mexican Americans and immigrant communities, has suggested to some researchers that the condition, one of the most horrifying to behold in the NICU, may be linked to farm work and exposure to pesticides or other agrichemicals.

Nikkol has had one setback after another: The reduction surgeries were not entirely successful, and portions of her intestines scarred over to form strictures—blockages—that make it impossible for her to digest food properly. At the age of two months she was transferred to Long Beach so that the medical center's famed pediatric surgeon, Visut Kanchanapoom, could try to salvage what little was left of her intestines, again with mixed results. Now she subsists on IV fluids, her liver and digestive system atrophying, her skin bronzed by the worst case of jaundice anyone here can remember, turning every part of her yellow, even her eyes. Attempts to feed her by G-tube—a tube surgically installed directly into her stomach—have failed. The food simply won't go through.

Nikkol's chronic illnesses, stemming as much from the multiple surgeries and other treatments as from the defect itself, have left her in constant pain and nearly immobile. The once tiny three-pound baby is bloated and overweight from the lipids pumped into her for nourishment; she now weighs fourteen pounds. Her neck has become so stiff from being in the same prone position while hooked to the oscillator that she can barely move her head. The months of injections, tubes, tests and procedures have taken another toll as well: She has developed a predictable distaste for being touched, except by her mother. This sort of negative conditioning is common among the chronics in the unit, but Nikkol's is particularly severe. She reacts violently to the slightest stimulus; even the sound of a nurse tearing a foil packet or the smell of an alcohol-soaked swab can cause a fit. Then the all-important oxygen saturation levels in her bloodstream—the "sats"—plummet, accompanied by flashing monitors and urgent alarms, and the nurses have to back off from whatever they are doing or risk having Nikkol asphyxiate herself out of pique and pain.

But with Sara Masur, Nikkol seems different. She softens, as she does when her mother pets her and tells her stories of a home life she has yet to experience and may never know. There is a gentleness about Sara, a calm, that seems to envelop the babies like a warm blanket.

The title "occupational therapist" does not begin to describe Sara's duties in the NICU, where her concerns focus less on immediate illnesses, on the current condition of hearts, kidneys and lungs, and more on the long-term development of the entire child. A better title for Sara might be unit visionary, or perhaps institutional conscience. She is there to think of the things that traditional medical thinking often omits and to ask the questions no one else is asking. It is Sara's job to wonder not just what will happen to the babies during their stay in the NICU but what will happen to them when they leave. She asks: What will become of these children when they reach their first or second or fifth birthdays? What can be done to make sure that the lives we save are as rich and rewarding as they can be long after the NICU is left behind? What, in short, are we doing *to* these children at the same time we're doing all these things *for* them?

These are questions that neonatology has only just begun asking. Until recently, little thought was given to anything beyond fixing the babies' immediate ailments, then discharging them from the unit in a month or two or six. The answers to these belated questions have at times been disquieting for neonatologists like Art, though he has been one of Sara's main supporters in the unit. What Sara and other pioneers in her field have shown is that the babies saved by the NICU can sometimes react to the world like abused children—abused by the very heroics that have kept them alive. Sara's job is to help minimize the negative side of medical treatment, and to help heal the unintended injuries that can come with it.

She fits this unique role well: There is no one else quite like Sara Masur here, her almost mystical approach to her job so at odds with a place dominated by machines and science and the laws of cause and effect. Most people who work in the NICU use clothing to announce their status in a dress code as exacting and rigid as the Marine Corps': The nurses have their floral-print scrubs and clogs or running shoes; the RTs favor dark blue, unadorned surgical scrubs; and the doctors (and would-be doctors) avoid being mistaken for nurses by—univer-

sally, as if it were taught in some first-year med school class—wearing
their stethoscopes draped around their necks like stoles, sometimes
with white lab coats flapping like wings, never buttoned. The lab workers have coats, too, though they button theirs. Sara Masur, however,
dresses like a parent, not a staffer. It sets her apart, which is fine with
her, because, though she is well liked and respected, her unconventional
views mean she can never really be part of the club. She is the sort of
person who uses her own money to buy special nipples and pacifiers
specifically designed for preemies. There would be none at all if Sara
didn't get them. Though they are readily available at the local chain
store pharmacy, the hospital cannot seem to find a way to purchase or
stock the type the preemies prefer. So Sara stashes her own bootleg supply in closets and drawers around the unit and passes them out like
contraband to nurses and parents she is working with, who never know
the source.

Now Art watches her slow, tender way of touching Baby Girl Hawkshaw, stroking her forehead with a firm, slow palm, so unlike the quick,
purposeful hands of the doctors and nurses. She whispers, "Hi, there,"
barely audible, her words part of the same rhythm as her stroking. Sara
always handles a baby as if she has nothing better in the world to do, as
if her office isn't as backlogged with paperwork and case files and bureaucratic detritus as everyone else's. The difference is striking.

So are the results: The nurses here are good at bringing their preemies along, very good. But it is Sara Masur they all seek out when even
they can't get a baby to suck or accept a nipple or swallow their food
without strangling themselves—simple tasks for normal babies, enormous hurdles for many preemies. It is Sara who finds ways to relax inconsolable drug babies. And it is she who works with the mothers
having trouble breast- or bottle-feeding, showing them how a finger
under a tiny chin or a slight change in posture or position can make all
the difference—and doing it in a way that encourages rather than dis-
courages mothers already feeling guilty and inferior. Sara draws the
toughest of cases. And almost without fail, she can cradle the babies,

massage them, cajole them, hold them in a certain way, and get them to feed, to suck, to swallow safely where others cannot. Sometimes she just holds her hands a few inches above a child's body, sensing without touching the trouble spots, the areas of pain, the centers of dysfunction—an empathetic gift she has had, she explains with some reluctance, since childhood. They feel warm to her, or cool, a tangible sensation that allows her to focus on the damaged areas. Such gifts do not really fit into the ultrarational world of medicine, which is why she seldom discusses them. She just quietly puts them to work, as she now does with Nikkol. Then, murmuring softly to her, she gently begins to massage the baby's neck, slowly loosening the knotted muscles and tendons. Nikkol tenses at first, then relaxes. No alarms sound.

"Look at that," Nikkol's nurse says after a while. "Her sats have actually gone up."

It is true. Nikkol Hawkshaw's vital signs haven't looked this good all week. If it were anyone other than Sara doing this, Art knows, the kid would be coding.

Now, Art tells himself, if they can just get that baby to eat, she may even make it to her first birthday.

11

Midafternoon arrives with faint sunshine slanting through the windows of Room 288, offering a gilded view of the Los Angeles basin's hazy sprawl. The unit is in a lull. The three o'clock shift change is approaching, one of the few times in the day when parents are asked to leave the otherwise open NICU. There are only a few family members around.

Dr. Mark Hachigan, a colorectal surgeon, began the day on the tenth floor and slowly made his way down through the medical center, floor by floor, patient by patient, conducting his rounds. At each stop, he read the chart, read the flow sheet, read the labs. Then he entered his orders and moved on to the next patient until he arrived here in the NICU, staring down at a baby born three months premature, his breathing sustained by a ventilator, his nourishment provided by IV.

Once again, Dr. Hachigan read the chart, read the flow sheet, read the labs. Then he just sat and stared at little Steven Hachigan, his premature son. The doctor is now in the patient's chair, and it is unbearable, for he is no more able to help or comfort his son, no more able to vanquish the fears and dread this place inspires than any other parent in the unit. He has just enough knowledge to scare himself.

"Why is he so slow to recover?" he asks aloud. He sounds humbled, despondent, his surgeon's air of invulnerability stripped away by the two-pound preemie in front of him, still on a ventilator after a month of care.

It had started on Halloween afternoon. He had been finishing up at work when his wife called and asked him to hurry home. Monique had gone into labor after rushing around town, getting their other son—Paul, a healthy three-year-old who was also born premature—ready for trick-or-treating. Monique had wailed all the way to the hospital, saying she didn't want a twenty-eight-week preemie, that he had to stay in, that she knew how bad things could be this early. But the drugs hadn't stopped the contractions, or her water breaking, or Steven's arrival. This was an order of magnitude worse than Paul's birth, which had been only two months early. His case was almost routine; he was in and out of the NICU in two weeks. There is nothing routine about Steven's case, however.

"He looks so much smaller than the others in the room, he's taking so much longer to improve," Dr. Hachigan says. "Why?"

"Every baby is different in here," Steven's nurse, Patty Rulon, reassures him. He has heard the words many times, but he can't bring himself to believe them—even though he has uttered similar sentiments about his own patients in the past. "Each one progresses at his own rate," Patty continues with deliberate certainty. "Steven will get there."

Patty has been at this long enough to understand this father's discouragement. Steven is what the NICU staff calls a "wimpy white boy," the insider's nickname for notoriously slow-to-recover white male preemies. Compared to girls and children of other races, they seem to have the greatest statistical propensity for lingering on the ventilator and for suffering ABs, spells of apnea (absence of breathing) and bradycardia (slowing of the heart). Indeed, Steven has been nicknamed the "King of ABs" by the nurses. The nicknames are affectionate, but even so, they are never spoken aloud when families are around.

"He's taking his time, but he is making progress," Patty says. "He's weaning from the vent slowly. He has no infections, he's tolerating feeds. He's just got to remember to breathe, that's all."

"Thanks," Dr. Hachigan replies, sounding less than convinced. He gathers his things and moves to leave. "It's the helplessness. I can't stand feeling helpless."

He stares a bit longer at his sleeping son. Steven sleeps constantly, it seems. There is a tape recorder inside the incubator, replaying the sound of the family talking, Paul reading a story—the familiar voices Steven grew to know in the womb, there to comfort him. There are toys and pictures and a sign one of the nurses put on the side of the incubator: "I want to go to the prom. Please don't forget my donut." The "donut" is a rolled-up washcloth shaped in a circle, which is placed under a preemie's head for twenty minutes every four hours or so, to keep the head from getting too flat and long. The ventilator forces babies to lie for unnaturally long amounts of time on their backs, and without the donut to relieve the pressure, the force of gravity can give their heads a misshapen, blockish shape. Patty reaches in and positions Steven's head on the cloth.

After a few more minutes, Dr. Hachigan walks slowly away, his shoulders slumped. Patty watches him go and says, "I feel bad for him. I mean, his son's going to be fine. This kid just needs time, and he'll be okay. But you try to tell a surgeon he just has to wait, that there's nothing he can do. For him, there's nothing worse."

Baby Girl Berger's father is standing over his daughter, sobbing, his chest heaving. The deadened calm on Harry Berger's face earlier, when he was in shock and talking to Lupe Padilla about his daughter's poor prognosis, has given way to a wild grief. Denise Callahan spots him through the window in her office. The nurse coordinator feels her chest tighten, but she cannot look away.

The limp, lifeless baby girl is being prepped by two nurses for transport by helicopter to Children's Hospital of Los Angeles. Children's L.A. offers the experimental treatment with minute doses of inhaled nitric oxide—a potentially toxic precursor of smog—to reverse the pulmonary hypertension that is making Baby Girl Berger's lungs fail. The new treatment has long been slated to become available in the Long Beach NICU, but red tape has slowed federal approval, making the transfer to Children's L.A. necessary.

This is the last straw for Harry. Alone and adrift, his wife in surgical recovery, he is unable to cope with the transformation of a picture-perfect pregnancy into a disaster in the space of a few hours. Was it just that morning that he was toting a camera around, hoping to capture the joyful moment of his daughter's birth? Now he is standing in the middle of Room 288 wailing—about the unfairness of it all, the awful possibilities that lie ahead for a baby who was dead for twelve minutes and who may never be able to say Mama or Dada or wave good-bye.

"These are the worst cases," says Denise with a sigh. She's been here almost as long as Long Beach has had an NICU. "The really sick pree-mies, I feel bad when they don't make it, but I can deal with it. They never really had a chance. But these full-term kids, they're supposed to go home. This isn't supposed to happen. When their parents lose it, I lose it."

She watches the father a moment longer as a nurse and the resident attempt to console him, with little success. Denise mutters, "Oh, this brings it all back. We had one like this fifteen years ago, I'll never forget it, a little boy, he cried and died. Heart defect. Nobody saw it coming. It was just me and the attending at the delivery. We worked on him for an hour, way too long, but we didn't want to stop. I could barely draw the epi, I was shaking and crying so bad. The doc was crying. The parents were crying. Everybody was crying. Fifteen years ago, and I can see it in my mind like yesterday. I hate cases like this."

She pauses, the memory a shadow moving over her kind, open face as she watches Baby Girl Berger's father, his face now buried in his hands. "But who knows, this kid today might be okay. You know, you work here, you can't help but believe in God, that there's something more going on here than what we do and what the doctors do and what the drugs do. I remember one time a baby coded in one of the step-down rooms. We did CPR, me and Jose, but nothing worked. No heart rate, no respiration, nothing. We called it, we stopped. I was starting to wrap her up to take her to the morgue. And she came back to life. Just started crying after the code was called. I'll never forget that one, either. And she did okay."

Several other nurses have come to see what all the commotion is about, and they nod at Denise's words. Someone mentions little Katia from a few years back, who weighed only fourteen ounces and was considered hopeless. Statistically, she should have been dead or profoundly handicapped. She's two now and is already reading, a precocious child who drops in for visits now and then with her mother, her only abnormality being her diminutive stature and her need for eyeglasses. Another old-timer remembers the twenty-six-weeker who had been left to expire in the treatment room, as was the custom back in the early seventies, when preemies of that gestational age could not be saved because ventilator technology was too primitive for such tiny lungs. Except this baby didn't know that. He cried for two hours, lusty and strong. They finally went in and treated him, put him on the ventilator, went all out to bring him around. He's a college grad now.

Everyone in this room has a story of the implausible, the miracle, the case that beats the odds. Maybe, Denise says, Baby Girl Berger will join the list.

The storytelling abruptly ends and everyone returns to work as Baby Girl Berger is wheeled out of the unit in a transport incubator, her father trailing after her, his face wet but his sobs quieted. Something about his silent, devastated look is worse to behold than the crying. Several of the nurses are wiping their own eyes as they leave.

A short time later, Kristine Hawkshaw is slumped next to her daughter's incubator. She is positioning a family portrait for Nikkol to look at: Mom, Dad, her stepsister and stepbrother, taken before Nikkol's birth.

The image of Kristine is particularly striking because of the contrast between her appearance then and today. She is thinner now, pale skin beneath long, dark hair, the striking model and dancer in the picture with the slightly spoiled look—the expression of someone who had known few hardships in life—stripped away and replaced by a more mature and far more haunted beauty. She has not eaten properly in months, her stomach erupting in an ulcer from the stress of swallowing all doubts beneath a dogged optimism that will not acknowledge the very real possibility that Nikkol might not make it home. Her friends, the neonatologists, even her husband, Stuart, have all gently tried to get her to accept that it is possible—only possible—that Nikkol could be too sick to pull through. She tunes out everyone but Stuart; when he suggests this possibility, she grows furious, accusing him of disloyalty, of being weak. Their fledgling marriage, younger even than the five-month-old Nikkol, is under siege.

"Nikkol is the strongest person I've ever met," Kristine always says, bludgeoning Stuart into silence whenever he tries to prepare her—and himself—for the worst. "She is going to make it."

It hadn't been all bad. Nikkol had been taken off the vent just a week ago. She was in the step-down room. Penny Jacinto had her in a swing. She'd loved it. But the "stim feeds"—small amounts of food given to stimulate her atrophying digestive system—had not gone well. A bilious, bloody backflow had come out of her stomach tube, and the feeds had been stopped. Then she had begun to show signs of infection: fever, desats, frequent ABs. Nikkol had to be put back on the vent and returned to Room 288. Kristine was devastated but refused to acknowledge it. "We've come this far," she said firmly. "We'll get through this, too."

Kristine is singing softly to her baby now. Nikkol seems relaxed after the session with Sara and has been looking up at Kristine, letting her mother stroke her hand and arm without pulling it away. This lets Kristine indulge in her favorite fantasy: What she would be doing if Nikkol were home. The image is very clear in her mind. She sees herself on a lazy Sunday morning, balmy air billowing the curtains. She is lounging in bed with the papers, a cup of coffee in hand, just watching Nikkol sleep next to her. That's all. Maybe she flicks on the TV, maybe not. Mostly she relaxes and listens to the sound of her daughter breathing. She could spend hours that way, given the chance. Most people take such things for granted, Kristine knows. But oh, what she wouldn't give to see her daughter lying there on her big old bed, snoring peacefully, life spread out in front of her like any other kid.

"We're going to do it, baby," Kristine whispers fiercely. "I promise you that."

While Kristine Hawkshaw is dreaming of life after the NICU, Lupe Padilla is holed up in her cluttered office, trying to grapple with life *in* the NICU. She is surrounded by mounds of patient files, reviewing cases, finishing summaries, taking care of loose ends between patients. A colleague looks in, hoping to have a chat with Lupe, but she takes in the piles of paper and says it can wait. As she turns to leave, she says over a shoulder, "Don't you hate all this routine work?"

Lupe shakes her head and calls after her, "This isn't the routine. The *babies* are the routine. This is the interruption."

Lupe is working on multiple tasks at once, feverish as usual. To her left is an unfinished memo on computer problems in the unit. On her computer screen is a partially completed e-mail concerning forty thousand dollars that an insurance company owes the neonatologists but won't pay. This will be the third notice she has sent; the financially failing company owes several million dollars to other doctors who are just as irritated as Lupe. Atop a pile of pink phone message slips is a note to call her husband, a pediatrician with far more regular hours than she. She'll save this one for later, when she needs a sanity-restoring talk about what groceries need to be picked up at the store and whose turn it is not to cook.

Instead, she dials an in-house extension and begins dictating a "History and Physical" for Baby Girl Berger. The H and P is the first report in any baby's file, documenting the birth, the mother's history, the baby's initial treatment, vital statistics, Apgar scores, treatment plan, prognosis. When typed up, an H and P is a two- or three-page affair, very formulaic and dry; spoken aloud, particularly by Lupe, it is a remarkable piece of oral history. She speaks into the phone with phenomenal speed, like a recording gone berserk and playing back double time. People who haven't heard her before drop what they're doing and gawk in amazement at the blur of words, run together yet completely comprehensible. "This is a full-term newborn female born to a thirty-three-year-old gravida one, para zero Caucasian mother by emergency cesarean section secondary to decelerations and terminal bradycardia." This sentence takes about three seconds to utter, less than half what a normal conversational tone would require. She does this from memory, with only a short note to remind her of grams and centimeters and other arcane numbers from the baby's delivery and resuscitation as she recounts, in the blandest, most jargonesque wording possible, the drama earlier that day in OR-9. She finishes the lengthy report in about two minutes. Somewhere else in the hospital, a stenographer will transcribe the call and deliver the completed report that same shift, so that it can be copied for the file for when Baby Girl Berger returns from her nitric oxide treatments after a week or so—if she makes it that far.

This efficient system of dictation and stenography has remained largely unchanged for decades, and Lupe, for one, would be content to leave it as is. But the age of the computer is upon the NICU, and a new system is coming on-line, one that is supposed to save time and money while greatly improving record keeping by digitizing the H and Ps, which currently exist only on paper. In the coming weeks, Lupe and the other physicians will begin putting these reports directly into the unit's new computer system, phasing out dictation for good. That will give the NICU an instant database on its patients, something Art Strauss has long wanted. But so far, the new system has proven to be painfully unwieldy: The complex forms embedded in the software have turned Lupe's two-minute telephone tornado into an hour-long hunt-and-peck exercise. The docs all hate it. They have no more time to give. This is the substance of Lupe's memo: The computer is supposed to be more efficient, not less.

She rubs her eyes. She cannot remember the last time she didn't feel tired. She used to think that a constant state of near exhaustion was normal, back when she was on call every third night as a resident and life revolved around work and little else. Maybe a movie now and then if she was lucky. She had no friends outside the hospital world. She even married another resident. If she had not literally bumped into a compatible, loving mate at the hospital, she undoubtedly would still be single—having time for intimacy outside the NICU with someone not in her line of work seemed a fairly remote possibility. Now she has a family, a large, comfortable home close to work, a housekeeper, an eleven-year-old daughter who is growing up independent and beautiful and whose life Lupe sometimes feels she is missing entirely while caring for other people's kids. She has call only one night a week now (most of the time), which should translate into a more normal life, but her existence remains just as dominated by work as always, if not more so. Since she, Art, Jose and Penny took over the practice, the administrative duties have piled up—all the committees, the meetings that never seem to stop, the fliers and marketing and promotions she has to puzzle over, things they never had to worry about when they were the employees instead of the employer. And all of it interrupts what she cares about most, the care of her patients. When she gets a week off, she is invariably in the hospital, trying to catch up, haunting the halls and snapping, "I'm not here!" to anyone who dares approach her with a request. Many nights, Lupe just crawls into bed and falls asleep by nine o'clock.

Now she feels a sudden urge to talk to her daughter, but gets no answer at home. Restless, she returns to look in on some patients and runs into an ugly scene between a nurse and the mother of a baby whose recovery from a heart defect and neurological problems has been halting at best. The mother is yelling at the nurse, who had simply asked her if she wanted to change her baby's diaper. Many mothers enjoy this chore in the NICU; it makes them feel a part of the care. And it gives the nurses a chance to observe how well or how poorly a mother handles her sick infant. But this mother, a difficult person under the best of circumstances, will have none of it.

"No, you change him!" she is saying angrily. "You're paid five hundred dollars a day. This is the Ritz-Carlton. Why should I have to change the diapers?"

Lupe knows this is an insecure woman who is attempting to exert control over the uncontrollable: a son who is not getting better very fast, whose heart condition has made him sluggish and unresponsive, and who will probably have lifelong problems. The mother remains in denial about her son's poor prognosis. She stays overnight in one of the family rooms, ostensibly to feed her son every three hours—feeding being one of his top problems—and instead watches television and refuses to come into the unit when her son is ready to eat. When she does come in, she turns the lights on and sings loudly in the nursery when the other babies in the room are sleeping, disturbing the routine, oblivious and quick to anger or weep if the nurses intervene at the disruption. She signs consent forms and then denies having given permission for important tests and procedures. She often seems more concerned by her own considerable medical problems than her son's. And she has a list of nurses and doctors she dislikes and who, therefore, she does not want to touch her baby. After three weeks in the unit, it is a long list and getting longer every day—much to the relief of those on it, though the logistics of staffing the room with nurses she finds acceptable is getting harder and harder.

"This hospital is just milking my insurance!" She continues to rail. "You don't want to do anything. I'm taking my son home!"

Lupe decides to speak up. She is tolerant of parents who carry on— God knows, the stress of having a baby in the NICU can make anyone crazy. But every once in a while a parent comes along who is so overbearing, so disruptive and so in the wrong that he or she needs to be reined in. Lupe accomplishes this in the quickest way possible: She simply calls the woman's bluff.

"Your son isn't ready for discharge, but you could go to another hospital if you're unhappy here," she says calmly. "We can help you arrange the transfer."

Lupe has said this in the blandest way possible, but the woman becomes panic-stricken. She begins to cry. "I don't want to go," she says, reversing field. "You can't make me go." She mutters something about having a friend who is a lawyer, but in the end she backs down. Which is all Lupe wanted to accomplish anyway.

"Thank you, Dr. Padilla," someone says after the mother stalks out. Lupe, meanwhile, makes an entry in the baby's chart asking for a consult with Sara Masur because the boy's poor muscle tone and inability to take in enough nourishment to sustain himself are signs of developmental problems, Sara's specialty. "This child's got a long way to go," she says, "so let's get him started."

A short time later, Lupe grabs a snack at the spare desk in the coordinator's office, where someone has put out a plate of cookies. "Heard you played hardball with Mrs. This-is-the-Ritz-Carlton," Denise Callahan says. "Nice going. Now *you're* on her list, too."

Lupe smiles. "As long as you tell her what she wants to hear, you're her favorite doctor," she says with a shrug. "I can't do that. I *won't* do that."

She glances at the door to the office, where the photos and cards to the unit get posted, and her eye is caught by a letter from the grateful, gracious parents of twins who were in the unit's care a few months ago. The letter thanks many members of the NICU staff, and Lupe reads it in silence: "You will always hold a special place in our hearts," it says. "You cared for our babies when we weren't able to, and shared our grief."

Most of the notes posted on the door come from the overwhelming majority of parents whose children do well, both in the NICU and afterward. They come with snapshots of once fragile children growing tall and strong, which are passed around like treasures. But this one letter stands out because it bears testimony to how the unit shines even in

times of tragedy: The first twin died of a massive brain hemorrhage after just a few days; the second boy was stable and doing better when the
family's HMO demanded he be transferred to their own facility, where
he died in the space of a week. Many members of the staff went to the
funeral and visited with the devastated parents on their own time; for
the parents to have written this letter, just a few short weeks after their
loss, amazes Lupe. She feels a surge of pride at being part of an enter-
prise that, even in times of heartbreak, helps people get through. It's
easy to forget in the onslaught of paperwork and meetings and endless
hours of work, but there really is only one routine here: *The babies, the
families, the caring are the routine,* she reminds herself. *Everything else is
interruption.*

The weary physician rubs her eyes yet again. Then she picks up the
phone and dials home. This time her daughter answers on the first ring.
Lupe has to clear her throat before she can say, "Hi, hon. Nothing special. Just wanted to hear your voice."

12

ROBERT ALLMAN FINISHES SCRUBBING UP, UNAWARE OF WHAT FATE has in store, hoping only that, at the end of this day, his family still numbers three. The secretary ushers him past the front counter; at the moment he is the only parent in Room 288. A nurse tells him where to go, and he hesitantly walks to the plastic box containing his son. The machines and alarms and activity all around him are almost too over-whelming to take in, as is Pure's straightforward explanation of the things being done to help the baby breathe, to protect him from infec-tion, to solve his low blood pressure, to keep him warm. The drugs and devices and techniques will all have to be explained again and again, by the nurses, by the doctors, by the social worker. No one expects him to absorb more than a fraction of what he is told: The same is done with all the parents, who are far more predictable in their reactions than the babies. At best, the doctors figure parents can retain about 20 percent of the information they receive at the outset. By the time they leave, how-ever, they will be reading the charts like pros, as conversant in the lan-guage of sats and electrolytes and PDAs as the nurses. For now, though, the concerns are simple: "He's going to be all right, isn't he?" Robert re-peats the question as if reciting a mantra.

The truth is, Baby Boy Allman should be fine. Twenty-eight-week-ers—a serious challenge fifteen years ago—are routine these days. Their problems have been so eclipsed by the micropreemies' that they actu-ally look big to the nurses who work this unit. Still, he is barely an hour old and there is a long road ahead, with many tests to be performed to determine just what ails him. And so the doctors and nurses are cautious when Robert questions them, offering variations of the same reply: *He's doing well. He's stable. We're watching him closely. His vital signs are strong.* These are the encouraging but neutral responses from professionals who know they must always nourish hope but never promise more than they know they can deliver.

"His color's good," a nurse says, and Robert nods, studying the numbers and lines on the monitor and trying to figure out what they mean. "Look at that hair," the nurse says, searching to give Robert something positive to cling to. "Just like his father's!"

For a long time, Robert stands quietly in front of the incubator, staring at the darkly bruised baby, the swollen eyelids and scratched, red skin livid beneath the fluorescent lights. The feet are so tiny they look like toys. He wants to touch the baby, but he is afraid. He remembers how his son seemed to turn toward him when he said hello in the delivery room, how he and Amalia had taken heart in the idea that they had already forged a connection with him.

Now Robert whispers "Hello" again. Nothing happens.

A moment later a technician pushes a bulky mobile X-ray machine into the room and calls out, "I'm looking for Baby Boy Allman."

The nurse who had been standing next to Robert filling out chart entries waves and says over here, and the big machine is jockeyed into place, clearing other incubators and respirators by inches. The technician extends the cantilevered arm that holds the X-ray projector, and Robert and the nurse have to step back out of range. "This is Baby Boy Allman, right?" the tech double-checks.

"His name is Elias," Robert says quietly as the hum of the machine clicks on and off and the briefly suspended bustle of Room 288 swirls back into motion.

PART II

DAYS PAST

"Take Two Aspirins and Call Me at Coney Island."

13

Paris, France
Near the Turn of the Twentieth Century

THE DOCTOR PACED HIS BELOVED HÔPITAL MATERNITÉ, SURVEYING the devastation. The sight of all those empty incubators and cribs, tiny sheets neatly tucked in, were unbearable—reminders of the legion of small patients he had just lost.

The epidemic had swept through the nursery with the subtlety of a sledgehammer, a swift and overwhelming respiratory infection that had ravaged nearly every infant in the unit in a matter of days. Most of the full-term babies had shaken off the infection in a week or so, as the doctor knew they would, but the flulike disease had overwhelmed the premature infants, helpless and mute in their incubators, their immature lungs and compromised immune systems easy prey for the invading germs. Most of the preemies had died; the few that had survived had done so at great cost, with brief lifetimes of pain and disability their inevitable legacy. Mothers wept beside the incubators, as the nursery lay quarantined, closed to new admissions until the infection burned itself out. All this in the world's state-of-the-art hospital for sick newborns, where the staff had boasted time and again of its success at saving infants others viewed as little more than stillborn. Until now.

What went wrong? Dr. Pierre Budin kept asking himself. *Where did I fail?*

It was no comfort to Budin, of course, but for most of human history, such a question would have been unthinkable. Indeed, in the not-too-distant past, the passing of Budin's premature patients would have been seen as an unalloyed blessing, for mankind had always relegated the infirm, the premature, the "weakling" babies to abandonment and death, the prevailing belief being that only the fit and the strong should survive, lest families, tribes and nations be burdened by the lame and the halt. Even with all the new century's gleaming accomplishments and promise, the care of sick infants lagged woefully behind other areas of medicine. In the recent past, obstetricians had ceased their ministrations as soon as the baby was delivered, while pediatricians remained unwilling even to examine a child before age two, leaving frail, sick infants to the advice and (sometimes toxic) nostrums of midwives, grandmothers and neighborhood busybodies. Caring for babies, doctors believed, was simply beneath them.

Modern medical advances had finally demonstrated that even the tiniest babies could be sustained in a man-made womb and given a chance at something close to a normal life. Backed by the French government, Pierre Budin tended to the smallest of the small, the sickest of the sick, in his Paris hospital with its advanced technology and techniques. But not, it appeared, advanced enough. And now he needed answers: Why had so many died? And what could he do to prevent the next epidemic?

The amazing thing is the answers that had eluded his predecessors for centuries *did* come to Pierre Budin, with world-changing impact—though whether the revelation was a slow one or a flash of inspiration, no one but he could say. But this much is known: As he watched the nurses move from patient to patient, feeding one of the babies that had survived the infection, cleaning and changing the child, then moving to the next, Budin decided what needed to be done: The nurses needed to wash their hands between patients. They needed to don a clean gown each time they touched another baby. Baby bottles and their contents needed to be sterilized, the milk kept on ice until ready for use. And the sick babies and their caretakers had to be kept isolated from the healthy infants.

This revelation, so commonsensical and obvious, was nothing short of revolutionary at the time. Indeed, many in the medical establishment bristled at Budin's insistence that his "special precautions" be scrupulously followed. Imagine, sniffed some, telling esteemed physicians to wash up like children called to dinner! His opponents might have won out but for Budin's timing: The French government, concerned by the country's high infant mortality rate and declining birthrate, seized on his ideas, financing his hospitals and clinics and even passing laws enforcing some of the doctor's notions. His methods slowly gained acceptance, first throughout France and Europe, then in the rest of the world. And with that, word spread of his other peculiar ideas: about measuring the weight and girth of premature infants in order to calculate how much nourishment they should receive; the use of something he called a "gavage tube" for depositing food into the stomachs of babies too feeble or small to suck; the use of tactile stimulation and oxygen masks when babies needed help breathing; and his fondness for the converted chicken-egg incubators pioneered by his mentor, Dr. E. S. Tarnier, and built specially by the curator of the Paris Zoo, for warming premature newborns, who have not yet developed the subcutaneous fat humans rely upon to maintain body heat. He created quite another stir with his fervent belief (against conventional wisdom but backed up by his own painstakingly gathered mortality statistics, another area he pioneered) that human breast milk was the best food for babies. Again, the old guard resisted his unconventional ideas—they preferred to administer cow's-milk enemas, testicular extract and various preparations of the toxic element mercury to deal with starving or cyanotic infants, rather than the battalion of wet nurses used at the Maternité. But Budin had glimpsed the future of pediatric medicine, and his ideas had a singular power: His babies lived, while the old guard watched their charges turn blue and die. Long after Budin himself slipped into obscurity, the practices he pioneered remain in use, at once vital yet taken for granted in virtually every hospital in the world that cares for babies.

The year was 1896, and without quite realizing it, Pierre Budin had invented the practice of neonatology—though it would not be known by that term for another six decades. It is Budin's legacy that, inside every modern NICU in the country, premature babies are weighed and measured and fed accordingly, with the same gavage tubes and calculations Budin pioneered. They are warmed in incubators, cared for in scrupulously sterile environments and, whenever possible, fed breast milk—a form of nourishment whose value was forgotten by the medical establishment for much of this century, though that tide turned for recent generations, once again affirming Budin's hundred-year-old research. The number of lives saved and made whole from the fruits of Budin's fateful walk through a disease-decimated nursery, the children who would live who otherwise would have died, the number of parents who celebrate first birthdays instead of laying flowers at small graves, are simply incalculable.

14

Before Pierre Budin's time, a quick and painless death for frail or ill babies was considered a natural and humane fate. Sick or deformed babies who clung to life after birth might be abandoned to the elements or killed outright, a merging of mercy and cool practicality. Any attempt to prolong such lives was considered a defiance of nature, an affront to the gods, even an assault upon the fabric of society. What happens in modern NICUs would probably be viewed as an abomination.

The epoch in which this sensibility prevailed was a long one, stretching from the ancient cave painters of southern France to the philosophers of ancient Greece, from Renaissance barbers with their leeches and bloodletting to Civil War–era surgeons with their nonsterile operating theaters and stogie-smoking onlookers. All shared the view that sick and premature infants were not meant to live, that they posed an unacceptable burden and that nothing could or should be done for them. Since the time of Hippocrates, it had been accepted as fact that, as the ancient Greek healer wrote, "No fetus coming into the world before the seventh month of pregnancy can be saved."

Hippocrates made that observation around 460 B.C., and conventional medical wisdom did not deign to revise his conclusion for more than two and a half millennia. The twenty-eighth week was an absolute cutoff. Very few at that stage survived, and none who were born earlier. Over the centuries, there was an occasional rare account of a smaller preemie who survived by being placed in a jar of feathers or some other primitive warming device, but these tales were mostly dismissed by men of science as hoaxes, exaggerations or the aberrant exceptions that proved the rule.

This thinking finally began to change late in the nineteenth century, when a few doctors in Europe began pioneering treatment of what were then called "feeble" infants. At first derided and dismissed, their cause was bolstered by a new societal pressure: the Franco-Prussian War. So many French soldiers had been killed in that conflict that the government had become concerned about the future of French civilization: An entire generation had been decimated. A decision was then made to try and save every baby, even ones who had once been considered beyond help. A new epoch in the care of premature and sick newborns had begun.

Soon laws were passed in France requiring mothers to bring their children in for regular postnatal checkups. New children's hospitals were built, financed by the government. Doctors and inventors began designing infant incubators, experimenting with everything from artificial wombs in which premature infants floated in warm water to room-sized heated environments that functioned like infant greenhouses. A League to Prevent Infant Mortality was founded and Pierre Budin put in charge, with his state-of-the-art clinic located next to the Luxembourg Gardens, near the seat of the French government in Paris. The birth of neonatology arose not so much from a humanitarian concern for children as from a practical consideration: France needed all the babies it could get in case it went to war again someday. Budin's radical practices were embraced not because he was a visionary and a man of compassion—though he was both—but because the government recognized that, if he delivered on his promise to reverse the deplorable infant mortality statistics that were making the country the shame of Europe, there would always be an abundant supply of cannon fodder.

And so specialized care centers modeled on Budin's ideas and those of a few other like-minded doctors sprang up throughout France. A corps of nurses specially trained in Dr. Budin's ways was put in charge of the day-to-day care of the preemies and other frail infants, rigidly enforcing the French doctor's rules for feeding, washing, care and isolation of infected infants. Visitors were discouraged, direct contact forbidden; even doctors were instructed to touch the babies as little as possible. Parents could only look through glass windows at their infants, as if they were rare hothouse flowers—which, in a way, they were.

Each of the new infant care centers was designed to address the three specialized problem areas for premature babies, identified by Budin in a groundbreaking book, *The Nursling:* preemies' temperature and chilling; their feeding difficulties; and the diseases to which they are prone, namely infections and respiratory distress. For the latter, Budin advocated piping pure oxygen into the sealed incubator, a wood-and-glass box heated by natural gas and a reservoir of warm water beneath the compartment holding the child. The oxygen mixed with the room air inside the incubator and provided a more concentrated form of the life-sustaining gas. Budin exercised caution with oxygen, using it only for resuscitation rather than as a frequently dispensed preventive. This, it turns out, was a key insight, though no one recognized it at the time as anything more than a cost-saving technique; tanks of pure oxygen were heavy, inconvenient and very expensive. Like his other views, Budin's ideas about oxygen were gradually adopted throughout the world as his methods and influence spread. There was no arguing with the results: Babies previously expected to die were not only surviving but thriving.

How word of these revolutionary changes spread is nothing less than bizarre. A Frenchman named Martin Couney, part physician, part pitchman, would later claim credit for saving countless babies from unnecessary deaths by transforming Pierre Budin's obscure theories into an international phenomenon. He accomplished this in the most unorthodox and, by modern standards, unseemly manner possible: by turning real preemies and their caregivers into carnival-like attractions around the world.

These exhibits, featured at world's fairs and international exposi-
tions, created a sensation, fetching the then-kingly sum of twenty-five
cents per visitor. In their most enduring incarnation, Couney's preemies became permanent attractions at Coney Island and Atlantic City,
along with Nathan's World Famous Hot Dogs and the diving horse of
Steel Pier. The Coney Island exhibit lasted for four decades.

Back in 1896, Couney was a young doctor working under Budin
when mentor asked student to take six of his latest incubators to the
World Exposition in Berlin. They featured air filtration, a humidifier
and an electric alarm bell that went off when the air temperature inside
rose too high—features still in use today. Doctors all over the world had
been tinkering with such devices, and Budin wanted to show off his
handiwork.

He may have wanted a scientific exhibition of high-tech equipment, not an entertainment for the masses, but Couney seems to have
had a flair for the dramatic: He decided to place actual preemies in the
incubator exhibition, watched over by a team of Budin's nurses. As
Couney would later tell it, a well-connected German obstetrician, persuaded by a letter of introduction from Budin, put the garrulous Dr.
Couney in touch with the Empress August Victoria herself, who soon
arranged for six infants to be provided by the Berliner Charité Hospital.
The doctors there readily agreed to the unorthodox display, concluding
that it posed little risk as none of the infants was expected to survive.

Showing his genius as a marketer, Couney laid claim to coining the
name of the exhibition—Kinderbrutanstalt, literally "Child Hatchery"—a concept that so enchanted the German public that the display
was soon overrun by tourists who paid a mark each to view the babies.
Kinderbrutanstalt went on to become the subject of drinking songs and
comic routines in Berlin's beer halls. Not even the vocal gymnastics of
the popular Tyrolean yodelers next door at the World Exposition drew
crowds like the Child Hatchery.

The Berlin exhibition lasted all summer. Couney and several other
doctors amazed the German medical establishment by graduating sev-

eral "batches" of preemies, bringing them all to a weight of five pounds or more without—Couney would later claim—a single death. Given his robust ticket receipts, Couney was invited to stage a similar display in London the following year, where he drew crowds as great as 3,500 a day. The staid British medical establishment at first refused to provide him with any babies, but Couney simply shipped a load of preemies in laundry baskets across the Channel from Budin's clinic in Paris.

The results were so impressive that England's respected medical journal, *The Lancet,* completely forgot its previous objections and gave the exhibit a glowing review. ("The incubators and the ventilating tubes are silvered," the journal gushed, "which gives them a bright and cheerful appearance, while the infants within look clean and comfortable, so that altogether it is a pleasant as well as an interesting sight.") *The Lancet* editorialized strongly in favor of adopting Budin's methods immediately; the premature infant mortality rate in London hospitals then hovered at about 40 percent, even for infants born only a month early. By contrast, the Budin methods put on display at Earl's Court were saving babies born far earlier and weighing far less—several as little as two pounds—and making the job seem almost routine.

The revolutionary nature of this cannot be underestimated: This was an era in which one out of ten *full-term* newborns died in the first year of life; Couney was doing nearly that well with his preemies. There were cases—rare ones, admittedly, but still remarkable for the time and technology—in which babies in his care weighing less than one thousand grams at birth survived, a feat that is considered far from routine even today.

After the London show, Couney's unusual exhibitions were much in demand and the heavyset, stooped French doctor became a familiar sight to thousands of visitors who came to see his babies and hear him extol modern medicine's latest miracle—"making propaganda for preemies," he called it. He, his incubators and his nurses traveled the world in style; the organizers of the Pan American Exposition in Buffalo in 1901 were so taken with his Child Hatchery that they built an enormous brick building for him with room for dozens of babies at a time. Lines extended far out the door for an entire summer, with many people returning again and again so that they could watch the babies' progress, a sort of episodic entertainment long before radio serials and soap operas.

The rousing success of Couney's shows led to neonatology's first misadventure: With such public interest, imitators were inevitable. County fairs, music halls and even Barnum and Bailey jumped on the incubator bandwagon. Barkers would stand outside the makeshift exhibitions, shouting, "Step right up and see the miracle babies!" (Their numbers included one handsome young man named Archibald Leach, who eventually gave up his job shilling for imitation child hatcheries in favor of a film career in the States—under the name Cary Grant.)

None of the imitators had Couney's credentials or cachet, however, and their less-than-premium commitment to quality was roundly criticized as abusive, unsafe and morally wrong. *The Lancet,* so enamored of Couney's showmanship, wrote a year later that his rivals should be shut down. "All sorts of persons, who have no knowledge of the intricate scientific problem involved, [have] started to organise baby incubator shows just as they might have exhibited marionettes, fat women, or any sort of catch-penny monstrosity," the journal editorialized. "It is therefore necessary that we should at once protest that human infirmities do not constitute a fit subject for the public showman to exploit. . . . Is it in keeping with the dignity of science that incubators and living babies should be exhibited amidst the aunt-sallies, the merry-go-rounds, the five-legged mule, the wild animals, the clowns, penny peepshows, and amidst the glare and noise of a vulgar fair?"

It was not always clear exactly how Couney's exhibitions differed in principal from the carnival shows *The Lancet* so deplored. Nonetheless, he apparently enjoyed an excellent reputation in the world of medicine, and he had no trouble persuading hospitals and obstetricians to send him babies to treat and display (it helped that he charged nothing for the medical care, paying all his expenses and staff salaries from ticket sales). The Children's Hospital in Buffalo first began caring for preemies by observing the nurses at the Pan American Exposition, then buying the used incubators from Couney once the fair closed. Julian Hess, the Chicago pediatrician who in 1922 built the first premature infant care center in the United States that wasn't attached to a fair of some sort, and whose texts influenced neonatal care in America for generations, credited Couney as a source of his inspiration. Thus was the science of neonatology brought from Paris to the United States, where Couney took up permanent summertime residence at Coney Island in 1903, expanding to Atlantic City a few years later.

For decades after that, Dr. Couney was offered more babies than he could handle, because few facilities existed that could match his expertise and capabilities. At the height of his popularity, Couney maintained two separate exhibits of preemies at Coney Island, and he continued showing his incubator babies until he reached his mid-seventies, just before the Second World War, with his last international exhibition at the New York World's Fair in 1939. At the end of his career, he estimated he had cared for more than 8,000 babies and that about 6,500 of them had improved enough to be sent home (a then-phenomenal survival rate of more than 81 percent). Couney's own daughter, a twenty-eight-weeker, was one of them. When she grew up, she became one of his neonatal nurses.

Thanks to the mass-marketing skills of Martin Couney, Pierre Budin's methods were adopted and followed throughout the world and observed religiously long after Budin himself was largely forgotten. As time passed, procedures were refined and incubators and other devices improved, but for forty years, the model Budin created and Couney promoted for caring for preemies remained intact.

Still, one problem seemed insurmountable: Even though the larger, better-developed preemies were surviving far more often than in the past, the same twenty-eight-week barrier to survival first enunciated by Hippocrates in 460 B.C. still held true in 1940: Babies born before the seventh month of pregnancy almost never survived. More twenty-eight-weekers were surviving than anyone had ever imagined possible, but there the progress had ended.

There was a simple reason for this: The immature lungs of babies born before twenty-eight weeks—and a substantial but gradually decreasing percentage of preemies born after that point—suffered from a deadly condition. Pathologists figured out the problem during autopsies: They found that the preemies' straining lungs became enveloped by a peculiar film of dead tissue and collapsed air sacs, a kind of membrane that sealed off the lungs' interior surface, impairing the tissues' ability to absorb oxygen and expel carbon dioxide. A name had been given this condition—hyaline membrane disease—but there was no treatment. Within two to three days of birth, the tiny air sacs collapsed, the surrounding tissue died, the hyaline membrane formed, and the baby could no longer take in enough oxygen to survive. Budin had solved the problems of warming and feeding premature infants and limiting their infections, but none of his methods could stop the self-destruction of the smallest preemies' lungs. As other ailments were vanquished, hyaline membrane disease became the number one killer of newborns.

For some preemies, everything had changed. But others might just as well have been born in the Dark Ages for all the good modern medicine could do them.

15

ART STRAUSS WAS BORN IN 1952, FOUR WEEKS PREMATURE. IT WAS HIS good fortune—and his curse—to be born in an era that had finally moved beyond Coney Island.

His birth to a nineteen-year-old mother and a father just returned home from the Korean War occurred in the midst of a new epoch in neonatology, an era in which doctors hit on the notion that using high amounts of oxygen to treat preemies would be a good thing. There was no such thing as too much oxygen, they assumed, only too little. Prevailing wisdom held that more oxygen would mean less hyaline membrane disease. And so, beginning in the 1940s, virtually all premature babies were given copious amounts of the lifesaving gas for days, weeks, even months at a stretch, whether they appeared to be in distress or not. This marked the first major deviation in four decades from Pierre Budin's long-respected and successful principles.

Art's parents never thought to question it, of course: They, like countless other parents, trusted the doctors to do what was necessary and right for their child. To be fair, that's what the physicians of the era believed they were doing. And so, without anyone really intending it, an entire generation of premature infants was treated as an unwitting laboratory experiment, subjected to an untested treatment with unknown long-term effects. The world was about to find out what unlimited amounts of pure oxygen could do to a premature baby—and to receive a painful lesson that preemies were not like any other human beings on the planet.

"The result was one of the worst calamities in the history of neonatology," Art tells his residents in a lecture he delivers every year, a presentation he calls "Therapeutic Misadventures in Neonatology"—part of his teaching duties as a clinical professor. "Ten thousand children were blinded because of a minor change in clinical practice, done without consideration of the possible consequences."

Ten thousand children blinded. Needlessly. Out of arrogance and ignorance. When he delivers this line in his lecture, he waits for the young doctors in training to grasp the enormity of this disaster—along with its humble origins. Oxygen, something used every day in every part of the hospital, had become a destroyer through misuse, causing a disease that could occur only in premature babies. And to make certain they understand its currency, he adds, "The epidemic peaked in 1952—the year I was born."

He says these last words wryly, as if to lighten things a bit, but there is an undercurrent of bitterness to his words. To this day, Art has persistent problems with his visual perception: He can't draw well, he says (the nurses who read his daily chart entries say, only half jokingly, that he can't write worth a damn, either), and certain three-dimensional constructs, such as his son's model airplanes, are objects of mystery. He attributes this to the medical misjudgments about oxygen use, which created an epidemic not just of infantile blindness but also moderate to severe visual impairment for thousands more—which perhaps explains his intense interest in medical misadventures and the ethical treatment of patients.

As a former preemie, Art has a personal stake in such matters, and though he was quite lucky compared to many other NICU graduates of that era, he still harbors anger at medical guesswork posing as valid science. That the victims of this misadventure should have been babies is especially disturbing to Art, who rejected working with adults during his medical training because so many of their ailments were due to their own bad conduct. This became painfully clear to him during a stint at a veterans' clinic, where he seemed to spend all his time trying, with little success, to counteract the effects of lifetimes of bad diet, lack of exercise, alcohol consumption, drug abuse and cigarette smoking. He hated it. Objectively, he knew there were many reasons his patients clung to their bad habits, even life-threatening ones, and that reining them in was beyond many. But in his heart, he still felt people were *choosing* to be ill. He found he had little sympathy for them and absolutely no desire to spend a career trying to heal them. They sucked up enormous financial resources because of their bad choices, billions of dollars in health care expenditures to treat smokers alone, something that troubled Art greatly.

But babies were different: They came into the world pure, blameless. He enjoyed working with them from the start, puzzling out their miniature systems and miniature problems, organisms so different from adult humans that they might as well be an alien species, with different reactions to drugs, germs, stimulation. To oxygen.

Art has no trouble justifying enormous expense and effort on a baby's behalf, the ultimate innocent victim. Which is why he is so troubled by neonatology's checkered past and why he is so adamant that young physicians in training be exposed to this side of his chosen specialty, whether they want it or not.

"Neonatology has a rather disheartening history on this score," he tells his residents. "There have been more therapeutic misadventures than we like to admit. And there may be more to come."

Thirty young men and women in baggy blue scrubs sit in a darkened lecture room in the bowels of the hospital and look quizzically at the NICU medical director. Some heads are drooping in the dimly lit room, with at least three residents fast asleep, crumbs from a tray of complimentary cookies spread across the tabletop in front of them. Doctors are notoriously poor historians of their own discipline. After all, if the subject is history, it has no practical utility in the examining room or operating theater, where only the latest of everything is acceptable. Young heads already overcrammed with new procedures and new prescriptions find absorbing Art's philosophical ponderings difficult. Attention wanders, soft snores can be heard. No one cares, though, least of all Art: Given a darkened room, a nonessential subject that will not be part of any subsequent exam and a large group of sleep-deprived medical residents, it is axiomatic that at least 10 percent of them will fall asleep. Seventeen years earlier, Art Strauss was known to do the same.

Those who are awake seem a bit confused, wondering exactly what they should be scrawling in their spiral-bound notebooks. The residents are used to hearing straightforward lectures on clinical practices and procedures, how to revive an asphyxiated baby or turn a defective heart into a serviceable organ—and they are used to hearing these presentations delivered in far more self-congratulatory tones than these surprisingly scolding words from a major player in the hospital hierarchy.

But then, the head of the NICU at Miller Children's Hospital has always been more gadfly at heart than administrator. The residents don't know it, but as chairman of the hospital's bioethics committee, Art more often than not takes the outsider's position, the nonestablishment view, tilting against the mainstream of his profession. He has regularly testified as an expert witness in medical malpractice cases, attempting to help distressed parents whose babies were harmed by deficient care in other hospitals. Contrary to popular wisdom about a legal system gone mad with enormous jury verdicts, Art knows most parents who take on powerful physicians and medical corporations have little chance of prevailing in court; he has risked alienating colleagues with his willingness to try to level the playing field. In his younger days, he joined the Physicians for Social Responsibility, with whom he promptly was arrested for trespassing while protesting nuclear weapons testing in Nevada. During a much-hyped press event celebrating the miraculous delivery of a preemie with a deathly ill mother, he stood in the back of the hospital meeting hall and pointed out that this "miracle" would not have been necessary if the mother had simply taken her medications and followed doctors' orders during her pregnancy. "What we're really celebrating," he said out of the corner of his mouth, "is gross irresponsibility and a half-million dollars of unnecessary medical expenditures, courtesy of the taxpayers." Art will never be a company man, his colleagues say, sometimes admiringly, sometimes not.

It is no surprise, then, that the misadventures lecture is Art's favorite. Through it, he can remind young doctors, who are otherwise entranced by the rosy recollections of medical pioneers and the marketers' celebrations of manufactured miracles, that most medical advances are, in fact, built upon catastrophe. Neonatology, for all the good it has brought to infants and their families, has a history of disasters. Learning from them, Art scolds his audience, is the only way to avoid new ones.

Fifty years ago, however, medical men weren't so concerned about learning from history. They wanted to *make* history. The post–World War II era brought a wave of optimism to America, a time when it was customary to think of great social, political and scientific causes as "wars"—and the medical world was no exception. Fueled by the development of new "wonder drugs," such as penicillin and the other modern antibiotics and immunizations, physicians and the general public found themselves embarking on a golden age of medical care. An unparalleled postwar economy made it possible, sparking the greatest building boom of medical facilities in the history of the world. Between 1946, when Congress passed the historic hospital-funding bill, the Hill-Burton Act, and 1949, more than one thousand new hospitals were constructed, thrusting the country to the forefront in medical care and achievements. Many of them included expensive new premature-infant care centers holding the latest technology—which, in turn, generated a need for more specially trained nurses and doctors to run them.

No expectation or pronouncement seemed too bold. It was assumed American determination and know-how would inevitably vanquish any enemy, be it the Axis powers, an invading microbe or the debilitating effects of premature birth. In the space of ten years, the United States went from a country where medical schools rarely mentioned premature babies—and the best facility for handling them was a summer carnival attraction at Coney Island run by an expatriate Frenchman—to a nation that possessed at least one dedicated premature baby care center for every state, with major urban areas hosting several. By the early fifties, New York City had ten such centers, precursors of modern NICUs.

During this medical building boom, two relatively unheralded developments occurred that would have unintended but fateful effects: The newly built hospitals incorporated the innovation of built-in outlets for dispensing oxygen at bedside, eliminating the need to wheel in heavy, bulky tanks; and the new Air-Shields company put postwar engineering and technical expertise to work and designed the Isolette Infant Care Station, which instantly became—and remains to this day—the standard by which all infant incubators are judged.

The Isolette changed the look of preemie care for good. Old incubators were heavy, opaque boxes of wood and metal with small glass windows through which little more than a baby's head could be seen. Their common lineage with zoo equipment was fairly obvious from their workshoplike appearance. Although they were heated, it was common practice to swaddle the babies so that all but their faces were covered, making even the smallest preemie look like a fairly normal newborn, even to the nurses and doctors providing their care.

The Isolette, however, was made out of clear Plexiglas, exposing the preemie's body to full view. The baby's sealed, transparent sleeping compartment had filtered, heated and humidified air—either room air or oxygen-enriched—circulating through it constantly. The Isolette included arm ports and rubber sleeves to allow nurses and doctors to reach inside, as if tending to some delicate lab experiment. Intravenous lines could be placed without even removing the baby from this technological wonder. Swaddling clothes just got in the way inside an Iso-

lette, and so babies were deposited in their incubators wearing only diapers, a practice that continues to this day.

As Dr. Robert Silverman, a pioneering neonatologist, has described
it, the new incubators had an unexpected effect: It was as if the doctors
and nurses were seeing preemies for the first time. The scrawny limbs,
pallor and heaving chests were suddenly and unavoidably visible
around the clock. The patients hadn't changed, but their debility was
visible as never before. And the impulse to do something about it,
something *more*, became irresistible.

That impulse was satisfied through research results that revealed
even healthy, asymptomatic preemies did not breathe in the same way
as normal newborns or adults. They experienced something called periodic breathing, in which their inhalation patterns and their sats var-
ied greatly over the course of an hour, cycling into and out of "normal."
Researchers at the Children's Hospital of Michigan found that piping
high concentrations of oxygen (70 percent as opposed to the normal 21
percent of room air) into the sealed incubators caused most preemies
to shift into more typical breathing patterns. (In this era, no one had
yet figured out how to use mechanical ventilation with infants; the incubators functioned more or less like the old oxygen tents used for
adults, a passive rather than active form of respiratory assistance.)

There was no real evidence that periodic breathing did any harm—
and no evidence that preventing it did any good—but correcting the
"problem" seemed to make common sense, and this study led to a nationwide change in medical practice. Instead of reserving oxygen as a
means of treating asphyxiated or cyanotic babies, as had been done for
forty years under the Budin guidelines, doctors began routinely pre-
scribing high doses and durations of oxygen for *healthy* preemies in order to keep their skin color pleasingly pink and their breathing in
regular rhythms.

It was here that the innovation of built-in oxygen at each bedside in
modern hospitals came into play: The new practice was simple, as the

oxygen was right there, just waiting to be turned on. And it seemed perfectly reasonable to go from giving the lifesaving gas to sick infants to providing it to *all* premature infants—what could be the harm? Those naked babies in the Isolettes immediately started looking better. Everyone was satisfied.

It was around this time that a once rare malady began to surface with alarming frequency in the eyes of premature babies: a scarring of the retina caused by abnormal, even wild, blood vessel growth. Over the course of twelve years, at least ten thousand children, most of them in the United States, succumbed to an epidemic of blindness, the end result of the most severe cases of the disease, then called Retrolental Fibroplasia—RLF. Thousands more would endure life with greatly impaired vision because of RLF, while untold tens of thousands would suffer from undiagnosed but real visual problems like Art Strauss's.

The most ominous aspect of this epidemic was that it seemed to be at its worst in the most advanced neonatal treatment centers in the country. It made no sense, or so it seemed.

In 1940, few people had heard of RLF. By 1950, it was the number one cause of blindness in infants.

The physicians and researchers trying to come to grips with the epidemic of blindness knew something had changed in their nurseries—something that was causing babies to lose their eyesight where it had never happened before. Countless possible causes and solutions were seized upon. Vitamin therapy, steroid treatments and other "cures" were not only proposed but widely adopted to fight the disease, each approach with its vociferous champions and critics.

Science was turned on its head. The supposed cures were put into use throughout the world *before* they were subjected to clinical trials, based upon claims of results in a mere handful of cases. This headlong rush to unproven cures usually was justified as a necessary leap of faith in order to "save the babies" or because "This is war!" It would be immoral to deny the treatments to infants while waiting for months or years of study, proponents would say. (Never mind the immorality of giving unproven cures to innocent infants after scaring unwitting parents into giving consent.) Scientific study could come later, it was argued, but now, we have to help these babies. The pressure was enormous: Action had to be taken.

The problem with this approach became apparent only years later, when the physicians realized that the cures were helping no one and curing nothing. In the case of steroid treatments, physicians were probably causing *more* instances of blindness and death among premature infants than would have occurred without the new "cure."

The one significant change the nurseries had undergone at exactly the same time as the epidemic of blindness and that now seems painfully obvious—the era's vastly increased use of oxygen therapy—was rejected out of hand as a possible cause for ten years. Pumping preemies full of oxygen, whether they seemed in distress or not, had become almost a religion. The link was finally made only because a persistent ophthalmology resident in Washington, D.C., sensed a connection and scraped together a grant to conduct a small study—over the objections of many other physicians. By simply scaling back the amount of oxygen given to one group of babies—providing it to them only when they were cyanotic and clearly needed it—and comparing the results to a control group of babies given routine, large amounts of oxygen during their weeks in the nursery, the study showed that blindness could be avoided almost entirely, with no ill effects on the babies. A mere resident had found the answer that had eluded the best medical minds for a decade: When it came to preemies, too much oxygen was too much of a good thing. The blindness epidemic had been manufactured by modern medicine.

Animal studies would later explain the mechanism behind this disease: The immature eyes of premature newborns react very differently from mature eyes because the blood vessels in the retina are still developing. After exposure to high levels of oxygen, they wither and vanish.

Later, the vessels grow back, but wildly out of control, resulting in scarring, retinal damage and blindness.

A national research study in 1954 confirmed the resident's groundbreaking work. Unexpectedly, the study's results showed that the concentration of oxygen was not the culprit in the epidemic; whether babies were breathing 30 percent oxygen or 100 percent was not a factor, as long as it was shut off as soon as the baby improved. The key was *duration:* on average, the shorter the time on oxygen, the better the baby's vision would be. This was welcome news, for it meant critically ill babies could be given short, lifesaving doses of oxygen, and still retain their vision. Preemies were no longer routinely given oxygen for weeks and months at a time and almost immediately, RLF again became relatively rare.

But the disaster was not over yet. State and local health departments were given guidelines that garbled the scientific findings. Physicians were told that RLF could be vanquished only through limiting the duration *and* concentration of oxygen. Not only were doctors told to return to the time-tested practice of giving oxygen only when babies were in respiratory distress, and for as brief a period as possible, they were told to limit the lifesaving gas to no more than 40 percent, less than twice the oxygen content of room air. To this day, it remains unclear why that added limitation became gospel, but it was adopted throughout the nation's infant care nurseries for the rest of the fifties and well into the sixties. Once again, medical practice was changed for no good reason—and once again, the consequences were dire.

The blindness epidemic receded. But now some babies who would have benefited in the first few days of life from brief treatments with high concentrations of oxygen, in the 80 or 90 percent range, did not get it—with tragic results. Deaths from hyaline membrane disease shot up 35 percent in the next five years, and the incidence of cerebral palsy and other brain injuries from oxygen deprivation also rose dramatically. One British research team, analyzing a decade's worth of statistics, calculated that each baby whose eyesight was saved because of restricted oxygen in this era cost the lives of *sixteen* other babies who were denied a lifesaving treatment. And no one could say how many other babies survived but went through life profoundly disabled—unable to walk or talk or feed themselves—because of oxygen deprivation and brain damage. One evil had been traded for an even worse one. It took another ten years for the erroneous and deadly restrictions to be eased.

These disasters shattered the confidence of many pediatricians, dampening enthusiasm for the research and science of premature birth. The nascent field of neonatology had lost its luster. The wild swings in the care of preemies, which would seem almost whimsical had they not led to such awful and unnecessary consequences, in the end benefited only one group: The trial lawyers had a field day.

16

I⊤ ⊤ook another ⊤en years, bu⊤ in 1963 every⊤hing changed and the modern practice of neonatology could at last begin. A young pediatrician who defied conventional wisdom and a national tragedy that reached into the White House combined to alter the landscape for good and put neonatology back on the cutting edge.

This leap in the care of preemies almost didn't happen, for neonatology had been stripped of its postwar optimism. The epidemic of blindness brought on by medical ignorance and arrogance had chastened researchers. And there had been other fiascos as well. Like the misuse of oxygen that blinded so many children, several other new treatments had been highly touted without scientific evidence, put into widespread use, then revealed to do far more harm than good—ranging from Epsom salt enemas that proved toxic, to the false belief that fasting and dehydration would help rather than hurt preemies by preventing edema and bowel infections, to the use of inhaled detergent mist and a miniature hyperbaric chamber that was supposed to mimic the pressures of being born in order to alleviate preemies' lung disease. These and other unproven treatments, as ridiculous as bloodletting by modern standards, were hailed as revolutionary cures in the years after the blindness epidemic. They were anything but. All were useless, and many led to illnesses and deaths that could easily have been avoided if the treatments had been tested first. Eventually, this history of disasters led to greater reliance on conducting studies and clinical trials before

putting new "cures" into practice, but the more immediate consequence was a reluctance among pediatricians to risk anything new.

But a young pediatrician in Toronto, Maria Delivoira-Papadopoulos, had glimpsed the future. A Greek immigrant, she came to her new
post at the Hospital for Sick Children fresh from battling childhood polio epidemics in her homeland. There she had become fascinated by the
mechanism of respiration, and she had become convinced that the
ventilator machines she had used to save older kids stricken with polio-
induced paralysis could be used to battle the number-one killer of
babies, hyaline membrane disease, which was then claiming the lives of as
many as twenty-five thousand infants a year in the United States and Canada.

Her superiors told her she was wasting her time. It couldn't be
done. And even if she managed to get an asphyxiated child onto a ventilator, it would be a cruel exercise, unnecessarily inflicting pain on
hopeless cases, for such babies could never be removed from the machine once started. The hospital could not sanction such a dangerous,
experimental treatment.

But Delivoira-Papadopoulos saw only the possibilities. She just
needed the right technology. The primitive ventilators then in use were
too crude. Their controls were not accurate or fine enough, and they
delivered air at pressures far too high to be useful with the tiny, delicate
lungs of infants.

So the pediatrician tinkered with the devices for many months,
modifying them like a mechanic in a garage until she felt they could
work with newborn babies without blasting their lungs apart. Even
then, Delivoira-Papadopoulos's superiors would let her work only on
infants who had been in respiratory arrest for many minutes, when
there was basically no hope left. Reviving the dead, she called it, when
she tried out her new machines on these lost souls.

Over time, however, she wore down her detractors and persuaded
colleagues to call her to the delivery room a little sooner if it appeared
they were going to lose a baby. If you've tried everything else, she argued, what have you got to lose?

And it finally happened. Summoned at the last minute when efforts to revive an infant through conventional means had failed, she ran up ten floors to put her new machine to work to try to save a child who otherwise would have been declared dead on the spot.

What seemed like folly, even sacrilege to her peers, worked. The new machine allowed a child to survive and eventually to go home with his grateful parents, a normal life ahead of him. Instead of just pumping oxygen into a baby's incubator and letting the child breathe it or not, doctors now had a machine that could breathe *for* the baby.

The device was awkward and inexact, intended for the sturdy, large lungs of adults, not the small, papery sacks of infants, even with the modifications. The device could easily cause a pneumothorax—a literal bursting of the lung, like an overinflated tire—and it did not easily imitate the rapid breathing patterns of newborns. But the concept had been proven, and researchers and medical device manufacturers immediately went to work adapting ventilator technology for the NICU. Breakthroughs came quickly after that, the way they always do once the label of impossibility is stripped away from a problem, like a runner breaking a record. Within four years, ventilators became standard treatment for the respiratory distress that was killing thousands of babies a year. By the seventies, an array of new machines built especially for infants became readily available, and a new technique for using them called "positive airway pressure," which keeps the lungs partly inflated at all times, never allowing a complete exhalation, kept hyaline membrane disease at bay by never giving the air sacs a chance to collapse and adhere.

Although there were many complications, including a new ventilator-caused scarring of the lungs called Bronchopulmonary Dysplasia and a tendency for the smallest preemies to become dependent on vents for many months or years, this gifted Toronto physician's untested belief in mechanical ventilation for babies hit the jackpot. It was not a perfect solution, and there still was a missing piece of the puzzle—the underlying cause of hyaline membrane disease remained

untamed—but a treatment had been found. The flawed lungs of preemies that had doomed so many for so long could at last be forced to
work by the new ventilators. Hippocrates' twenty-eight-week barrier
was finally cracked wide open.

Solving the last part of the preemie breathing puzzle, the cause and prevention of hyaline membrane disease, would take many more years.
But the path to that solution began in another hospital in 1963, just a
few months after that first baby was saved with a ventilator. This time,
however, advancement came though a life lost rather than a life saved.

On August 7, 1963, during a very long, very hot season of world crisis and tragedy, Patrick Bouvier Kennedy was born, the third child of
the young president and his wife, Jacqueline. Normally, this would have
been cause for national celebration, but Patrick had arrived six weeks
prematurely.

By today's standards, his birth at this stage of his mother's pregnancy would hardly count as premature. At just over four pounds, this
thirty-four-weeker would have better than a 98 percent chance of survival. But in 1963, his prematurity—and, more important, the critical
deficiencies in his small lungs—posed a formidable challenge to doctors. The Kennedys were told he had a fifty-fifty chance of making it.

Babies in respiratory distress who were very small or very early
were still simply allowed to gasp and die after delivery. Maria Delivoira-
Papadopoulos's successful ideas about ventilators were still largely unknown and untested, and it would be years before they made their way
into the Massachusetts hospital where Patrick Kennedy was born. Until
then, hyaline membrane disease would kill more babies in the first days
of life than any other cause. And the president's son was destined to be
one of them.

Patrick Kennedy died of respiratory failure after only thirty-nine
hours of life, John F. Kennedy beside him in tears, holding the infant's
small hand through a portal in the incubator.

The baby's death was a national tragedy, though it would be

eclipsed only three months later by an assassin's bullets in Dallas. Yet the helplessness of the medical profession to heal even the child of a president had a profound effect. Patrick's fate propelled a tidal wave of research that eventually led to the discovery of surfactant therapy, a treatment that, while not a cure, has made death from the effects of hyaline membrane disease rare and all but unheard of in babies of Patrick Kennedy's size and maturity. Scientists identified the substance that was missing from premature lung tissue, found a way to create it in the laboratory, then figured out how to get it inside ailing lungs. Then years of trials and study followed—there would be no repetition of the RLF disaster this time, no putting the treatment into use without solid proof that it worked and that it caused no harm. Surfactant became one of the nation's most heavily studied and reviewed treatments before the U.S. Food and Drug Administration finally approved it in 1990.

The problem of preemie's breathing seemed largely solved. Years on the vent became months; months became weeks; weeks evaporated into days. Ventilators and surfactant therapy changed everything in the NICU in the last decades of the century, just as Pierre Budin had changed everything at the century's beginning.

Once again, though, there would be a caveat, a hidden cost, the type of unintended consequence that comes with even the most wondrous developments. The ability to rescue small preemies with surfactant, ventilators and oxygen has been a lifesaving blessing for many, but for some, an old enemy has returned with a new name: A disease called Retinopathy of Prematurity is now rampant in the nation's NICUs among the micropreemies. It is the principal cause of visual impairment and blindness in infants, and it most often strikes babies who can survive only through long weeks and months on the ventilator—babies who would have perished a decade ago but who now are surviving in great numbers. Art Strauss calls it a new epidemic.

In the 1950s, they called it something else: RLF, the disease that blinded ten thousand babies. The long bouts of oxygen therapy needed to save ever-smaller babies has brought back an old enemy with a new name. It is now understood that the disease is much more complex than previously thought: Exposure to light, vitamin deficiencies, certain drugs used in the NICU (including the one needed to close PDAs) and diminished oxygen and nutrition to the fetus before birth all appear to increase the risk in preemies of visual impairment and blindness, along with exposure to too much oxygen in the NICU. Ophthalmological exams are routine in the nation's NICUs now, and cryotherapy and laser surgery to preserve vision is fairly common among smaller preemies, making the picture far less bleak than in the 1950s. Still, hardly a day goes by in the NICU in Long Beach without doctors finding at least one more child suffering some form of the disease—the price, it seems, of survival. It remains the number one cause of blindness in infants.

17

C~INDY~ W~ASSON IS STANDING VIGIL BY THE INCUBATOR IN~ R~OOM~ 288.
She has been there almost nonstop for the past three days, the hardest
three days of her life, transfixed by the struggle being fought before her
eyes inside a small plastic box: her daughter's struggle to live.

It is fall 1979, a time of transition and upheaval in the world of
medicine—a time of amazing advances, but also of stubborn reliance
on outdated methods by the old guard. When Cindy went into premature labor, she did not receive new drugs that could have stopped the
contractions, or that could have stimulated development of the baby's
lungs in case her labor could not be halted. Instead, she was sent home
and ordered to drink alcohol once an hour, a discredited method intended to halt premature labor that does more harm than good. Much
later she would wonder if her obstetrician didn't know any better, or if
he simply thought, incorrectly, that a baby as premature as Cindy's had
little chance of survival. Five years before, maybe, and certainly ten, he
could have been right about that. But by 1979, he was dead wrong.

At the time, Cindy had no way of knowing that, however, and her
mother dutifully plied her hourly with screwdrivers. Cindy had never
been much of a drinker. The cocktails made her sluggish and sick,
even as the contractions grew worse. She gave birth the next day, September 28, though Lindsay Wasson was not due until Christmas Day.
After Lindsay was born, she was rushed immediately to the NICU at
Long Beach.

Cindy was struck by the enormous contrast between her obstetrician and the energetic, bright, young neonatal staff who awaited her in the new NICU and exuded such confidence as they handled her impossibly tiny child, smaller than her husband's hand. She sensed immediately that she had landed in the right place: high-tech, efficient, gleamingly new.

The doctors and nurses were quietly, tactfully, horrified by her obstetrician's decisions. They were kind, they were solicitous. But Cindy also saw they spoke the language of modern medicine, a language of restrained expectations when it came to twenty-eight-weekers like Lindsay—babies who, in 1979, regularly were being saved but still posed formidable challenges. Cindy found little comfort in the noncommittal comments offered when she asked about her daughter's prognosis: *She's stable. We're doing everything we can. So far, so good. Only time will tell.* They talked about all the bridges she would have to cross before going home. No one made any promises.

It was hard for Cindy not to imagine the worst during those terrible days. The first time she touched her daughter—there had been no opportunity even to *see* her in the delivery room, and it was hours before she even knew whether she had a girl or a boy—she was so afraid she might damage the fragile little body that she simply stroked the bottom of Lindsay's foot. Even the clumsiest touch could do no harm there, she figured. But the little girl withdrew her foot as if her mother had used a red-hot poker and began to howl a catlike scream, high and awful. It sounded as if every alarm in the place went off as the baby's sats plummeted, and her heart rate shot off the scale. Cindy was terrified. Even when the nurses tried to comfort her by saying it wasn't her fault, that blood had been drawn a few minutes earlier from that heel, leaving it sore, Cindy couldn't stop crying. Her first touch, and she had caused her baby pain. What kind of future did that promise? What kind of mother would do such a thing? The already terrible weight of guilt she felt at Lindsay's prematurity, the feeling that somehow it was all her fault, became unbearable as she maintained her vigil.

Then, on the third day, a young man in rumpled blue scrubs shuffled into Room 288, his shoes tucked inside disposable paper booties, a surgical mask hanging limp from his neck. He stopped in front of Lindsay's incubator and began flipping through the chart. Cindy watched him suspiciously, not knowing if he was a doctor, a respiratory therapist or an orderly. He had no name tag. He looked pale and exhausted, his shoulders rounded, the posture of a man who has been up all night. Cindy was about to ask, just who are you, anyway, when the man cocked his head and looked at her with a tired smile on his unshaven face.

"So, are you going to bring Lindsay to our Bunny Bash in April?" he asked. "That's the reunion we have every year for all the preemies who graduate from the unit. You really should plan on coming. It's a blast."

Cindy could not have been more shocked if he had pulled out a banjo and started strumming. His words took a moment to register; then their import finally struck her: This man was the first human being to talk to her about the future, the first person who seemed to take it as a matter of course that there would *be* a future. She found herself returning the man's smile and saying yes, darn right we'll be there, and suddenly feeling quite certain it was true.

Like the newborns themselves, small things can take on enormous significance in the NICU: a baby's coo, a tiny hand squeezing a mother's finger, a negative blood culture . . . a kind word. That one optimistic comment was all it took to turn Cindy Wasson's dread into hope. The tired young man in the scrubs became Cindy's mainstay, the person she and her husband most often sought out when they needed to know what had happened and what was to come. By the time Lindsay left the hospital six days before her official due date, Dr. Jose Perez, then the unit's newest neonatal fellow, had become the baby's godfather.

Cindy has adored Jose Perez ever since, watching him over the years as he evolved from a young neonatologist in training to a respected attending physician, a doctor who prides himself in turning nevers into maybes, in being the last doctor to proclaim a baby sick enough to enter the NICU and the first to pronounce a baby ready to leave it. Jose had the good fortune to enter a branch of medicine at its most exciting moment in nearly a century, a time when the future once again seemed full of promise, offering the prospect that every baby, no matter how small, could have a fighting chance. New frontiers were being blazed. There had been enormous progress since that first ventilator had saved a baby in 1963, a virtual revolution in how premature babies were viewed and dealt with. There was a new fervor and inventiveness—a kind of medical *right stuff*—that was, in its own way, as exciting and novel as the space program had been in the sixties. That's how it felt to be a neonatologist coming up in this age: Neil Armstrongs for a new generation, giving families hope who, in years past, would have had none. When Jose began his training, he was told twenty-six-weekers almost never made it. When his fellowship ended, a twenty-six-weeker who did not survive the delivery room was the exception. Nationwide, that translated, into tens of thousands of lives saved, almost in the blink of an eye. Lindsay Wasson was one of the first babies of this new era, born on the cusp between the old ways and the new, a time when new medical advances and lessons learned from past blunders combined to save children who had never before been saved.

And Lindsay did go to that Bunny Bash in April, as Jose Perez had suggested. Cindy Wasson made sure of it. And Lindsay didn't just go to that one celebration in 1980. She went back year after year, right up until she went to college.

"Isn't she gorgeous?" Jose announced each time, showing off his blushing goddaughter to all the parents of newborn preemies who wondered if their two-pound pumpkins would ever overcome their shaky starts and blossom. "She's on the volleyball team. She does theater. She gets straight As—well, almost."

You could see the hunger in the eyes of the parents in the room, whose babies still struggled with breathing and seeing, who took twice as long to walk and speak as their full-term neighbors, who sometimes seemed so far behind they could never catch up. These moms and dads devoured Lindsay with their eyes, then saw the picture of what she had looked like in her incubator—just like their own children had looked— and they knew then that it was all worth it, no matter what.

"This is what you have to look forward to," Jose told them one year. They can see there is passion in his voice, and certainty—the steadfast look of a man who loves his work, who continually marvels at the small lives he nurtures and protects, who has glimpsed the ineffable inside his patients, a spirit, a will to live, that at times exceeds the sum of the treatments and drugs and surgeries in ways that continually surprise.

"This is the pot of gold at the end of the rainbow," he said, his arm around Lindsay. "This is the blessing you all deserve. Believe it."

It was 1993 when Jose spoke of that pot of gold. Lindsay Wasson was fourteen by then. If showing off his former patient to new preemie parents remained one of his great joys as a neonatologist, this year was also shadowed by an aspect of the job he despised. The political jockeying and internal strife that have become all too common in the world of medicine reached a critical mass at Long Beach Memorial that year, and threatened to rip his beloved NICU apart.

Jose was older, rounder, grayer then, his bushy hair thinning, his youthful idealism tempered by years of reality, though his core of optimism remained intact. He had been joined by Art Strauss, Lupe Padilla and Penny Jacinto, along with a number of other doctors, all of whom worked as attending physicians, having moved from ranks of residents to neonatal fellows to experienced neonatologists with reputations for excellence. That progress was the root of the problem now gripping the NICU: The attendings felt it was time they took the next step forward, becoming partners in the practice rather than mere employees. But working out such a transition with their medical director proved harder than they hoped.

The director of the NICU, a talented physician and shrewd businessman by the name of Dr. Houchang Modanlou, was in his eigh-teenth year at the helm of the unit. Modanlou's skill and vision had transformed a small and unremarkable infant care department into the world-renowned and groundbreaking model for neonatology that greeted Cindy Wasson in 1979, the largest in the West at the time.

Physicians and hospital officials from all over the world flocked to Long Beach in those heady early years to tour the unit, cameras in hand, jotting notes, studying the new layout and step-down rooms. Visitors wanted to know about the unit's revolutionary concept of entrusting nurses and respiratory therapists with greater authority than tradition-ally given, as well as the unit's commitment to the then-new nationwide push for "regionalization"—the notion that a few large NICUs serving an area were better than many small ones. Large NICUs with many pa-tients could quickly build expertise for physicians and nurses, which meant better survival rates for the babies, and they could better afford state-of-the-art neonatal facilities as well. Given its leadership in all these areas, Modanlou unabashedly—and correctly—described his NICU as a nationally recognized center for neonatal care and research.

But it had always been *his* unit, and this became a source of resent-ment for the attendings who had long worked there. They had helped make this unit what it was, too, they said, working extremely long hours for salaries they believed to be well below the going rate.

The attendings' dissatisfaction was compounded by the enormous upheaval in medicine that had begun at the start of the decade, not only with the march of scientific advances but also the transformation of the economics of medical care. The government cut back its cover-age of the poor and aged (a significant part of the patient population in urban Long Beach); insurance companies were going broke; mega-medical corporations were gobbling up practices and patients on a daily basis, keeping themselves alive through endless, restless expan-sion—a tactic Wall Street endorsed by bidding up stock values, until the companies who championed it began to collapse under their own weight and stopped paying their hospital bills.

Most of all, the rise to preeminence of health maintenance organizations as the engine of patient care fundamentally transformed the way medicine was practiced and paid for—or not paid for, as is often the case. Doctors who once got whatever they asked for began receiving pennies on the dollar from HMOs. Hospitals were forced to cut deals with these companies, offering bargain rates with no room for profit. Some bills would not be paid for months, even years—or not at all.

During this crunch, one bright spot could be found, at least in Long Beach: The Neonatal Intensive Care Unit became the cash cow of the children's hospital. While many other departments operated in the red, the NICU's earnings helped save the nonprofit hospital from bankruptcy. In part, this was because federal and state programs that pay for infant care are more generous—and more timely—in their reimbursements than many HMOs. Low-income patients, once a drain on the hospital budget, were now coveted. Another factor keeping many NICUs in the black was an unwillingness on the part of most private insurers and HMOs to cut care to babies as they did to other patient populations; that could have generated too much heat, too much negative publicity for an industry that wished to avoid regulation at all costs. HMOs and insurance companies know the only thing legislators find harder to resist than their lobbyists is a grieving mother in front of a microphone, tearfully recounting how her baby would have survived if only some coverage or other hadn't been denied. The insurers nibble at the edges of neonatal care, they push for early discharges or transfers to less intensive settings, but by and large, they ante up.

But the economics of neonatal care were creating a new problem: After years in which the preference was for concentrating sick babies in a few large, regional NICUs, suddenly almost every hospital wanted its own neonatal unit, no matter if it was small, no matter if training and equipment were rudimentary compared to the big regional centers such as Long Beach. Hospital chains and the HMOs that own or contract with them wanted to keep billings in-house, keep the profit margins high, keep the costs down. They couldn't cut care to babies, so instead of cutting off the flow of money, they tried the next best thing: to take over the practices with a wave of mini-NICUs intended to siphon off the easiest neonatal patients, the ones who required only routine care (and were highly, quickly profitable), while leaving the costly, time-consuming problem cases to the big, established NICUs.

This led to a new era of "de-regionalization"—not the best idea for patients or for the quality of medicine but a great way to make a quick buck. Hospitals own the physical space and equipment of an NICU and provide the nursing and support staff, but the physician groups who actually run the medical care in neonatal units are separate corporate entities; many neonatologists in the smaller NICUs are employed by conglomerate medical groups that sell and purchase tens of thousands of "lives," as patients are called, in a single transaction. The competition became so intense that some of these medical groups began ordering their younger neonatologists to sleep in hospital closets or to spend the night out in their cars in the parking lot, hanging around rival hospital nurseries trying to get referrals, trying to get a foot in the door of another unit, trying to muscle in on established practices.

All this meant more competition and fewer patients for each NICU. By 1993, times were tough at the Long Beach NICU. Plans to remodel the unit for the new millennium had been scuttled for the moment for lack of money. Raises were small, the hours longer than ever. A number of attendings had left. It was against this backdrop that Jose, Art, Lupe and Penny finally began formal talks with Modanlou about joining him as partners.

For a time, it seemed that this might happen, but eventually the negotiations broke down, the barrier to agreement seemingly less over money than over decision-making authority, the four attendings would later recall. A meeting to settle matters ended badly, with the normally reserved Penny Jacinto storming out, her colleagues following. A short time later, Art, Jose, Penny and Lupe were gone.

The four doctors, unable to practice in their old NICU because Modanlou had an exclusive contract, joined another physicians' group and scattered to other hospitals, a difficult, harrowing time for them. But they retained their staff privileges at Long Beach and launched an appeal to the hospital bureaucracy, making the novel argument that the hospital's exclusive contract with their former employer restricted their ability to practice medicine in their chosen specialty, something the hospital staff rules supposedly ensured. The four former attendings were now asking that the Long Beach NICU be opened to all doctors qualified to practice there.

Months passed as this proposal wound through the labyrinth of hospital committees and departments. No one knew who would prevail in the end, although a hint came at the annual children's hospital staff meeting four days after Art, Jose, Lupe and Penny left the NICU. Art, then vice chief of staff of the children's hospital and in line to become chief, was voted NICU Physician of the Year during the annual hospital staff meeting. He received a standing ovation, the only award recipient to be honored in such a way at the normally sedate affair.

The neonatal nurses, meanwhile, were in an uproar. The day the four attendings saw their last patients, a dozen or more nurses put their own careers on the line by donning black armbands in protest. This was not an easy thing for them to do, but these nurses had long enjoyed a special bond with the departed physicians. The tough working conditions had helped break down the walls that normally exist between doctors and nurses. Everyone considered themselves underpaid. Everyone worked hellacious hours. And these nurses grew up professionally with Art, Jose, Lupe and Penny, surviving their early years on the job, the practical jokes and endless double shifts. They respected one another's skills and trusted one another's judgment. They had become almost like family.

No such bond existed between the nurses and the doctors who took over in the unit—just the opposite. The collection of neonatologists and nurse practitioners hired as replacements were thrust into a busy NICU with which they were not familiar, handling patients and proto-cols new to them. Many of the nurses made it clear they were dissatis-fied with the change in personnel.

The families of babies coming into the unit in this period had no way of knowing about any of this, of course. The Long Beach NICU is very good at being open with parents about the care of its small patients, but when it comes to the sort of political battles embroiling the unit in 1993, medicine remains very much a closed world, its inner workings and conflicts hidden from public view. Although the neonatal nurses expressed concern to superiors, the hospital's official position was that quality of care in the NICU had not diminished, and that the new neonatal staff was doing just fine.

But then the nurses did something seldom seen in the insular society of medicine: A large group of them went public, picketing several times with placards saying, "Bring Our Doctors Back." They picketed at the children's hospital staff meeting where Art received his award and, a month later, at the hospital board of trustees meeting. More important, the local media was tipped. Newspaper reporters picked up the story, and the embarrassing headline in the *Long Beach Press Telegram,* "Physician of the Year Among Four Dismissed," troubled the hospital administration enormously. Negative publicity is no small matter for an organization whose existence relies greatly on charitable donations and community goodwill—and on the perception that quality care is a prime consideration.

Whether this public display tipped the scales in the end is unclear—the nurses and the doctors they supported seem to think it was a factor, perhaps even a decisive one. The medical staff of the hospital soon sided with the four departed attendings on the staff rules question, and the hospital administration ended its practice of granting exclusive contracts for NICU operation. Art, Lupe, Penny and Jose were back in. Modanlou soon left to take charge of the neonatal fellow training and research program run jointly by the University of California at Irvine and Long Beach Memorial—with his primary offices at the university medical center rather than at the hospital. The new neonatologists and nurse practitioners he had hired soon left as well. Competing in the open unit became difficult as the local obstetricians and pediatricians sent most of their patients to the neonatologists with whom they were most familiar—Art, Jose, Lupe and Penny.

But the crisis was not quite over. The four attendings had never been in business for themselves. They had always had the comfort of a paycheck. They had griped and chafed, but they had enjoyed security. Their duties had been 100 percent medical, stripped of the administrative tasks, the politicking, the annual budget wars. So instead of striking out on their own, the four attendings had decided to join a large medical group headed by a pioneering neonatologist, Louis Gluck, once a champion of regionalization, but now one of the proponents of mini-NICUs. Though some of Gluck's tactics concerned them, the four neonatologists believed they could join the group on their own terms. They were promised eventual partnerships, with Art slated to become director of the NICU. It was also understood that the four of them would stay together at Long Beach no matter what. Art gave up his chance to be chief of staff at the children's hospital to stay with the NICU he loved.

But the promises remained unfulfilled. Time passed, but there were no partnerships for the foursome, even though the Long Beach NICU quickly became one of the most profitable in Gluck's group. And Art was never made director. Instead, Gluck installed another member of his group to head the NICU—just temporarily, it was said. The hospital administration was said to be upset about the protests and accompanying adverse publicity; things would have to cool off a bit before Art would be accepted at the unit's helm. The four attendings reluctantly agreed and waited, relieved, even elated, to be back doing what they loved, in a place that felt like home. But the temporary director lingered for one year, then two, then more, with no end in sight.

Then a new bombshell was dropped: Gluck wanted to sell out to a nationwide chain of neonatal units, the Florida-based conglomerate Pediatrix, which had been buying up practices all over the nation. If the deal went through, Art, Lupe, Jose and Penny would not stand to profit at all from the sale, for they had never been made partners. This was particularly galling to them because the crown jewel in the sale, what made it so attractive to Pediatrix, was their Long Beach neonatal practice. They would be merely employees of the new company, which they feared could place them wherever it wished. Large bonuses were promised, but there was some troubling fine print in the offer: There were no guarantees that they would stay together, stay in Long Beach or even stay with the company beyond ninety days.

As they pondered this offer and the life changes it would bring—they had seen other doctors throw in with large corporations only to find little joy left in their work—the four neonatologists found out that they had been misled. The Miller Children's Hospital administration, it turned out, had no objection to Art Strauss directing the NICU. Dr. Mel Marks, head of the children's hospital, stunned them all when they finally went to him to hash things out about why Art couldn't run the NICU.

"I never knew Art *wanted* to be director of the NICU," Marks told them. Personally, he said, it sounded like a great idea. He asked for a written proposal.

With that cleared up, the four of them opted out of the sale to Pediatrix, forming their own company, Neomed. Theirs would be a different sort of medical partnership, one where the partners still did the bulk of the medical care, still did night call, still got their hands dirty— in addition to the endless meetings, committees and other administrative responsibilities they would have to take on. They nicknamed themselves the Four-Headed Dragon, a wry reference to the fact that they would all have an equal say in all major decisions. There would be a director, but no more monarchy in their NICU, no more hidden agendas—just an unwieldy, happy democracy.

Yet they were still vulnerable to takeover attempts. Their fight against the exclusive contract had opened the NICU to all neonatologists with staff privileges. But for their fledgling partnership to be viable, they would have to get most of the babies coming through the unit, or they would not be able to cover their costs. They could not ask the hospital for an exclusive contract—that would have been the height

of hypocrisy after their own revolt. Yet if other doctors started siphon-
ing off their referrals, they might end up breaking up anyway.

Then Jose hit on an elegant solution. They would propose a new
hospital staff rule with the primary purpose of enhancing the quality of
care in the NICU, but with the secondary effect of giving them domi-
nance over the unit. It would require twenty-four-hour coverage of the
unit by attending physicians for all babies requiring intensive care. Residents and fellows could help, but there would have to be a full-fledged
neonatologist there around the clock. If a doctor admitted a critical-
care patient, then that doctor or a board-certified neonatologist working with that doctor had to be there, twenty-four/seven.

The medical staff of the hospital voted in the change. It was a win-
win situation for the medical center, a great marketing tool. Other
neonatologists around the country, however, considered it lunacy. Such
an arrangement is unheard of in the medical world. Attendings are the
royalty of the profession; they get to go home for dinner and leave the
long nights and lumpy cots to the doctors in training, the reward for
their own suffering when they were residents and fellows. Indeed, in the
past, Art, Jose, Penny and Lupe had basically run the unit at night as
residents and fellows.

But changing that long-held tradition was the price of dominating
the NICU without a contract, while upgrading the level of care. In Long
Beach, the attendings would be down in the trenches forever; their pay-
off would be security, not restful nights and long vacations. They knew
competitors would be discouraged from ever setting foot in the NICU
with that bylaw in place. Any outside neonatologist who tried to come
in would have to start out small, struggling for referrals against the
well-established, highly regarded Four-Headed Dragon. Maybe a newcomer would be able to get a baby or two—but then what? It would not
be cost-effective to keep a neonatologist in the unit around the clock
just to care for a couple of babies. Most doctors with hospital-based
practices make their money by seeing many patients in a day, moving
from patient to patient, department to department, even hospital to

hospital in a single workday. That's how you rack up billables, something you can't do if you are stuck in the NICU all day with one baby to watch. The financial losses of such an operation would be staggering, as round-the-clock coverage works financially only with dozens of babies to treat. And so the new bylaw gave the Four-Headed Dragon everything an exclusive contract could offer, without the contract.

There was some speculation that Pediatrix still might send in an army of neonatologists and go to war against the four upstarts, for such a large company had the resources to take a loss in order to get established. But time went by, and the onslaught never came.

"We're home," Lupe declared, when she unpacked her boxes in what had been Dr. Modanlou's office. It appeared she took special delight in taking his space, even if she had to share it with another doctor. The secretary the former medical director had employed was also long gone, the anteroom she had occupied outside Lupe's office turned into a separate office for the NICU's clinical nurse specialist. The spacious suite of offices was now more like a college dorm, crowded and messy.

It didn't matter. They had won the NICU war. The unit was theirs. For the time being.

PART III

GETTING BETTER

"Some kids just decide to live.
Whether they're supposed to or not."

18

Progress Report:

Allman, BB

Day of Life: 15

Days in NICU: 15

Condition: . . . . Downgraded from stable
to critical

Diagnosis: . . . . PDA, RDS, possible bowel
obstruction

Plan: . . . . Surgical consult requested

Dear Elias,

Mom is kind of sad tonight. I know there are always ups and downs in life but I'm always hoping for more ups when it comes to you.

Your stomach has been bloated since yesterday. They did an X ray and didn't find anything wrong except for maybe gas or bowel distention. Hopefully that's all it is. You got another blood transfusion and other meds to help your lungs.

Elias, you're in my prayers. I pray that you will grow stronger and be healthy and happy. It's hard for me to see you when I know

you're in pain or uncomfortable. I know you are strong and will

grow stronger every day. Mommy just has to be strong, too.

Lupe Padilla puts her hands inside Elias Allman's incubator and gently squeezes the boy's stomach, her long fingers encircling her tiny patient. She clucks her tongue and says reprovingly, "Not good, not good."

Elias's abdomen has swollen several centimeters compared to just a few days ago—an ominous sign. He has actually lost weight; he has a wasted look, his ribs prominent despite the bloat. He has not been able to tolerate food. All attempts to get half-strength breast milk past his ventilator tube and into his stomach via gavage feedings have failed. Most of it comes right back up, and the little that does stay in his stomach makes him bloated. Today, the sausage shapes of his bowels are clearly visible beneath the drum-tight skin of his distended belly, and they are getting dangerously swollen. He is pained even when his stomach is gently wrapped with a tape measure, part of the rigorous stats taken each shift that graph his urine output, blood pressure, sats and every other imaginable measurement of human existence.

"He's very loopy," Patty Rulon, his nurse this shift, remarks. This is NICU-speak for the loops of bowel visible beneath the skin, a very dramatic and visible sign of abdominal distress. "It's gotten worse since this morning. His girth's up an inch. His blood gases are crappy, we had to go up on the vent. And he hasn't stooled in five days now."

"Why aren't you pooping, baby?" Lupe asks the child, her tone mock scolding. Elias is unaware, of course. He is in a sedated sleep, his ventilator pumping away, filling and emptying his lungs. Most babies can't tolerate the breathing tube down their throat; without sedation they spend all their time and energy feebly trying to tear it out.

Elias had been weaning from the machine, at first progressing well, but now his ventilator settings are higher than ever in order to keep his sats where they should be. An analysis of a blood sample that measured its oxygen and carbon dioxide content—a test performed regularly on every baby in Room 288—showed too little oxygen and too much carbon dioxide, the "crappy gases" Patty spoke of. Too much carbon dioxide makes the body acidotic, an altering of its normal acid-alkaline balance. This can damage organs and, if not corrected, can even be fatal. The underlying reason for this is that, despite surfactant treatments, Elias's lungs appear more damaged than ever: He has atelectasis, a condition in which pockets of air sacs in the lung's lining collapse, impairing the body's exchange of oxygen for carbon dioxide. Any hope that he would make a quick exit from Room 288 has been dashed by this setback—and now by his stomach problems.

Lupe continues her examination, musing out loud, ticking off a mental checklist: "X ray was clear, no obstruction, no NEC."

Necrotizing Enterocolitis, the intestine-destroying bane of preemies, which at onset can look a lot like Elias's condition, has been ruled out—for the moment, at least. A panel of three X rays of the abdomen taken from different angles, called an obstructive series, found no evidence of this dire ailment, nor were any abnormalities detected in the structure of the bowels that might be creating a blockage. Abdominal ultrasounds revealed nothing, either. The problem with NEC, however, is that it is notoriously difficult to spot in its early stages.

"Glycerin suppositories didn't loosen things up," Lupe says. "What about rectal stim?"

In medicine, jargon is often used to describe simple matters. A nosocomial infection is a disease contracted in (or more precisely, from) the hospital—a concept so scary (and so common) it has to be given a name few laypersons can pronounce, much less understand. An idiopathic condition is a lofty way of saying: We have no idea what's making you sick. And rectal stimulation is nothing more than a thermometer dipped in lubricating jelly, then poked around in the appropriate place to dislodge anything that might be stuck. Meconium—the hard, black material that forms in a fetus's intestines before birth—can sometimes form a barrier in the intestines. Healthy newborns purge this from their systems almost immediately, but a sick preemie may be too weak to pass it. The blockage lingers there for days, growing worse, silently at first, then with increasingly ugly symptoms as the digestive system backs up behind this dam.

"I tried," Patty says. "Nothing. You thinking what I'm thinking?"

Lupe nods. "Yup. I think it's a meconium plug that's too far in to get with rectal stim. Time for some Roto-Rooter. Let's call in the surgeon."

19

A FEW STEPS AWAY, JULIE FRANCE, THE NURSE COORDINATOR FOR THIS eight-hour slice of the NICU day, is hunkered over a battered Rolodex as if it were a patient on life support, feverishly calling up off-duty nurses at home, laboring to fill six openings on the next shift. It is not going well; no one is answering, probably because they know the nurse coordinators always call around this hour when they come up short. Her next step is to turn to the nurses she *can* corner—the ones already here—and order them to pull extra duty. This is called "mandating" overtime, though its victims have other, less polite names for it as well.

"This," one of Julie's nurses says in weary disgust, jabbing a thumb at the NICU coordinator's office as she hurries past, "is why we need a nurse's union here. I'm on my second double shift this week. And the hospital administration could give a damn."

"Don't blame the messenger," Julie's tired-sounding voice answers from the cluttered, closet-sized nurse coordinator's office. "Even though I know you will."

The problem Julie is facing is one of simple arithmetic: The unit is swamped with babies, and more babies require more nurses. Not more doctors, but nurses, the backbone of the NICU. Julie needs more than she's got. It happens this way now and then, random increases and droughts, rather than steady streams of patients, that move from the low thirties (mandatory days-off time) to fifty or sixty babies or more (angry-nurses-working-too-many-hours time). There have been seven admissions during the shift so far. And there are more babies cooking "in back," as the NICU nurses call the labor/delivery area of the medical center, including a set of extremely premature quadruplets. Julie can only hope the OB is successful in halting the mother's labor; she has neither the room nor the staff for four more tiny, sick preemies. Everyone is already working overtime and double shifts and crawling into work at three in the morning just to keep the lid on what's already here. Resentment—along with union talk—is at an all-time high. And Julie, whose job can be best envisioned as part of a game of tug-of-war—the rope part—has to work it out.

The nurse coordinator may have the toughest job in the neonatal unit. For eight hours, she is indispensable. She is expected to solve every problem, fill every need, find every missing thing, person or paper and settle every dispute and complaint on her watch, while also setting up the next shift for her successor, making certain there are enough nurses for the patients long after she has gone home. The importance of this job cannot be overestimated: Neonatologists may dictate each baby's care, but they spend only a few minutes a day with any one child; the nurses actually care for the babies, spending eight or twelve hours at a pop with just one or two of them. The coordinator is their leader, matching each nurse's skills to each baby's needs, looking over their shoulders, staying on top of the progress or problems of every infant while all the while holding together an often fractious, disgruntled, proud group of professional women. Julie's job requires the skills of an air traffic controller, trail boss, politician, counselor, diplomat, juggler, warrior, salesman and den mother, in addition to formidable nursing skills, an easy rapport with the docs, and a preternaturally tough hide. Julie France is one of the handful of people at the heart of the NICU, the small cadre of natural leaders who hold the place together through a mixture of charm, stubbornness and force of personality.

Those skills are being tested today. This is the worst crunch Julie has seen in a while, not because every bed is full but because so many of the babies are critically ill. Her boss, Chris Lombardi, the manager of the unit (whose own job encompasses the duties eight people once handled before downsizing gutted the budget), has been frantically trying to get some new hires to relieve the pressure, but the latest crop of new nursing grads—uncharacteristically—has been fleeing the unit in droves. It's too much for them: There are heart babies, gut babies, Down Syndrome babies, septic babies, four-hundred-gram babies so small they seem to vanish inside their Isolettes, babies whose problems are as yet unknown. Neurosurgeons, cardiologists, epidemiologists, ophthalmologists, gastrointestinal specialists and radiologists have been tromping into the unit at twice the normal rate to deal with these kids. And there are shell-shocked parents wandering around everywhere, refugees camped out in the unit's two small family rooms, drinking vending machine coffee, waiting for the reality of their situations to sink in, asking the same questions over and over.

"Why is this happening?" one woman in a hospital gown says to no one in particular as she trudges wearily toward the door of Room 288, her arm bristling with bandages, bruises and a disconnected IV port. Julie glances up at the new mother who gave birth less than six hours ago to a pale, still daughter with a package of defects called hypoplastic left heart. This is often a dire condition with no easy fix, and the woman is shaking her head, speaking softly as she drifts wraithlike past Julie's office. "What did I do wrong?" she wants to know. Julie starts to get up, but another nurse comes over and takes the woman's arm, leading her toward her baby and murmuring, "You didn't do anything wrong. Things just happen sometimes." The mother shakes her head, guilt being a common reaction that is not easily defeated by rational argument. The temptation is always there to say, if the baby is sick, it must be someone's fault. And the easiest person for a mother to blame is herself. Julie can see it in her posture as she steps painfully through the unit: overwhelming, stabbing, irrational guilt. Most every parent experiences it—except, it seems, the ones who ought to.

Julie sighs and returns to her Rolodex and telephone. As she dials, she cradles the receiver between her chin and shoulder, freeing one hand to hold and rock a sleeping infant. The baby, wrapped in a striped flannel blanket with a blue knit cap pulled down to his eyebrows, is nestled in the crook of one crossed leg. Julie had scooped up the baby from one of the small, less intensive rooms, where he was lying in his crib bored and crying. She saw that he'd been fed and changed and realized the reason for his wails: He was lonely. The nurses working the room had feedings to do, meds to draw; they were too busy to pick him up (or any other baby in the room) just for the sake of holding him. Babies need to be held, but sometimes there is no time. Which is why parents are encouraged to visit any time of the day and stay as long as they like—and to hold the medically stable babies, feeding them, changing them, bonding with them whenever and however possible. This poor boy, however, has not been so lucky: his parents have been no-shows. So Julie snatched him up for a good half hour of plain old cuddling while she works the phones and goes about her other duties.

Handling babies is not really the coordinator's job, and her office is not intended for patient care, but it's something she and her fellow coordinators like to do when they have a chance. There's nothing medically wrong with the baby; he's a "rule-out sepsis" case, an otherwise normal full-term newborn admitted with fever, poor sats or some other symptom of a possible infection. These are the most common, least sick, biggest babies in the NICU, and the staff's job is to identify and treat the infection or rule it out and send the baby home. The possibility of this baby boy having an infection has already been ruled out after three days of cultures failed to grow anything, but he's still here because of a history of drug abuse in the home. And because he is healthy and vigorous, he needs to be held far more than the preemies and sick kids; indeed, he demands it. Julie coos to him and wonders what his future holds in store. Holding him will be the most pleasing thing she does all day.

Julie dials another number, gets no answer, hangs up, starts over. Flip, dial, hang up. She has been doing this nonstop for the last twenty-five minutes without finding a single body to snatch from a day off.

Straining to hear, Julie tunes out the bang and thrum of the NICU scrub sinks shutting on and off and the two separate conversations going on around her in the claustrophobic coordinator's office, the occasional barb hurled her way. She must endure the resentment of the overworked nurses, as tangible in the air as the rancid smell wafting from the aging can of caramel popcorn sitting in a corner—a gift from a large and insolvent medical group that not even the hungriest med student would eat. She even manages to put out of her mind the thousand-yard stare she spots on the young, dark-haired woman scrubbing her hands raw just outside, one of the newer moms on the unit, Allman. All the nurses know Elias because of his unusual middle name: Jedi, a concession Amalia finally made to her *Star Wars*–obsessed husband. Julie has never, in thirteen years of NICU work, gotten used to that universal look of confused anguish she glimpses on Amalia's face, the look of a parent who thought her child was on a steady upward journey, only to find out that things just aren't that easy with preemies. Julie makes a mental note to check on Amalia Allman first chance she gets. She knows the new mother will be getting bad news as soon as the scrub sink's three-minute green light flashes on and she walks in to see Elias.

"Pick up, pick up, pick up," Julie chants, returning her attention to the telephone and the answering machine she hears droning on the other end. It's hopeless, she decides. Time to put on the witch's hat and start ruining people's days.

"I hate mandating overtime," she says absently to the baby in her lap. He opens his eyes briefly to squint and yawn up at the woman holding him, then goes back to sleep with a small grunt. "But I *have* to. I have six holes to fill."

Every coordinator has her own coping mechanisms to get through a tough shift: Julie's latest is a toy she got at a burger joint with her son's Happy Meal, a miniature baby from the cartoon series *Rug Rats*. With a squeeze, the toy's tinny voice lisps, "A baby's gotta do what a baby's gotta do." Julie turns it on whenever something really ticks her off; it's been played a lot today.

169

As she shoves the Rolodex aside and begins scribbling something on her patient status list—the notes she'll use to brief the next coordinator at shift change—the unit secretary buzzes her. "Got two more coming," Jo Ann announces, looking through the window between the front desk and the coordinator's office, her mischievous smile only widening when she hears Julie groan. "Now, *don't shoot the messenger,*" she says mockingly. "You got a Down's baby with heart trouble in Garden Grove and a drug baby in Cerritos. They want transport as soon as possible."

Before Julie can turn to the blinking hold lights on her telephone, a nurse working the Fat Farm sticks her head into the coordinator's office: "One of our young mothers just threatened to stomp Gloria's ass."

Julie and her baby both look up. Gloria is one of the older nurses in the unit who prefers to work the less intensive rooms. Julie asks, "Which mother would that be?"

"The sixteen-year-old, you know, the one who went into early labor after she was kicked in the stomach. We all thought it was the boyfriend who did it, but turned out he's the best of the bunch, that the girl's own mother kicked her—that one." The other nurse shrugs, resigned to the fact that while the NICU can work wonders on babies, it is mostly helpless at fixing the broken families some of the kids have to go home to. "Great family," the nurse says, unable to resist some private sarcasm out of earshot of patients. "Into kicking, I guess. Just thought you should know."

The nurse leaves, and Julie sighs yet again. She calls Art Strauss in to take the transport calls, then walks off to play the role of peacemaker, the rule-out sepsis baby still cradled in one arm, sleeping. She'll see if she can put out the fire before security has to be called. And then, when the dust settles, she'll get to order a few more nurses to stay late. As she walks down the hall, a tiny, tinny voice speaks from her pocket, over and over: "A baby's gotta do what a baby's gotta do. . . ."

20

"HE NEEDS A WHAT?" AMALIA ALLMAN ASKS WHEN SHE FINISHES scrubbing up and enters Room 288. Her face crumples at the news awaiting her.

"He needs a surgical consult," the nurse repeats. She continues talking, explaining that it isn't so bad, not an actual surgery at all, just a sort of supercharged enema, but Amalia can't make sense of anything after hearing the word *surgical*. She looks at the bloated belly, at the look of pain that keeps flitting across her sleeping child's face, and she begins to cry.

"It's not really a surgical procedure," Patty repeats, finally getting Amalia's attention by looking directly into her wide brown eyes welling with huge tears. "The procedure is called 'rectal irrigation.' Our nickname for it is 'Roto-Rooter.' The surgeon shoots water up into the bowels and loosens everything up. It cleans everything out, which is really what we need to do to make him feel better, before the blockage in his bowels gets worse."

Amalia manages a smile; that doesn't sound so bad. "Is it painful or just uncomfortable?"

"I think just uncomfortable."

"So I can watch?"

"Well . . ." Patty hesitates. She knows even benign procedures can look pretty horrific in the NICU. Even Lupe Padilla gets squeamish at Roto-Rooters—the same doctor who blithely intubates babies and plunges needles into their chest gets the willies over this one. Patty tells Amalia, "You may not want to stay for this one."

Amalia wipes her eyes and gazes lovingly at her son. He is barely visible beneath ventilator tubes and IV lines and the half-sized diaper that still looks too big. His face is obscured and his belly terrifyingly large, veined and bilious, as if someone has etched those tubular shapes into it. But when Amalia looks at Elias, she sees something else, the tiny fingers and their perfect little nails, the brushy blond surf-dude hair that looks as if it came right off Robert's head, the way his toes curl when she touches his foot. It takes effort at times, but she can half-close her eyes and see only what's beautiful inside that incubator.

"No. I want to stay," she says. "He needs me."

"Okay, then." Patty smiles approvingly at the new mother, youthful in appearance but grounded, mature, coping. "I guess a few weeks ago, you never in your wildest dreams expected to be in here waiting for a surgeon to Roto-Rooter your son, did you? It can be overwhelming here at times."

Amalia nods. "The first thing you need to understand," she agrees, "is, when you have a preemie in the hospital, life as you know it is over."

Like many families with babies in the NICU, the Allmans learned this lesson just as soon as the initial shock had faded and Amalia stopped hemorrhaging from Elias's bruising delivery. They soon found that most of a preemie parent's waking day is spent getting ready to visit the NICU, driving to and from the NICU, calling for updates from the NICU, thinking about visiting the NICU or actually visiting the NICU. The visits, the briefings from the nurses and doctors, the poring over the chart, the vigils next to Elias have become the focal point of the Allmans' existence. Nothing else seems to matter.

Along the way, they have become well versed in the language of the place and know all its many acronyms: RDS, NPO, PDA, NEC. They read Elias's chart like a John Grisham novel. They know the drug Indocin is being given to close the PDA channeling too much blood into Elias's lungs. They know surfactant treatments were given twice to ease his RDS—his respiratory distress syndrome. They know NPO means nothing by mouth, a term they desperately wish to see stricken from their son's chart. His bulging belly will not permit it, however. Still, Amalia marches dutifully to the "pump room," as she calls it, a private area with two electric breast-milk pumps in it where preemie moms express the precious nourishment into plastic bags, which are then marked and frozen in the NICU. Amalia is doing this at home as well. When a baby is ready, the breast milk, at first watered down but later given at full strength or even fortified with formula, is fed by gavage tube. Later, bottles will be used, when the suck, breathe and swallow reflex appears and the baby has the strength to sustain it, and then actual breast-feeding can be started as well. The stockpile of little Baggies for Elias is mounting up, a sad reminder that he is far from well.

The intimate knowledge of NICU science and culture that now seems second nature to the Allmans did not come easily. It seemed at first that they could never get used to the place, to the machinery, to the deathly ill children, to the expressions of fragile hope and despondency on the faces of the other mothers and fathers. What does a fragrance-line account executive manager for Calvin Klein know about mothering a lab experiment? How do you get used to the remoteness of your own baby, Amalia wondered, so unlike the chubby, full-term infant we expected to hold and kiss and smell? This was motherhood by long distance, as if she hadn't carried him at all, and Amalia is the kind of person who needs to touch, to forge a connection with hands and hugs and closeness. It was agony to be told that holding her baby would hurt him, that talking too loudly would hurt him, that touching him too much would hurt him. Later, they were told, it would be okay later. Soon. But not now. It was agony, the worst time of Amalia and Robert's life.

Dealing with people became difficult. The well-intentioned phone calls from friends and family soon became unbearable, and after a while they stopped picking up. You could only explain what had happened so many times before your head started to shoot off. People didn't know what to say. Some called and offered congratulations, as if Elias's arrival had been like any other birth, which Amalia and Robert knew wasn't right. Others offered condolences, as if it would have been better if Elias had never been born at all or, worse still, as if he were dead. And that *really* wasn't right. Yes, they had some wonderful, supportive friends. Their parents were great. People would just show up at the door, hand over a cooked meal and say, "Here, call us if you need anything else," then leave, sensing that now wasn't the time for visits. That really was helping. Still, they felt isolated, alone. It seemed as if no one really understood what they were going through. None of the pregnancy books, none of the exercises or Lamaze classes or visits to the obstetrician had remotely prepared them for this. *My God, when we went to pick a hospital,* Amalia railed to herself, *all we were interested in was the furniture, the food, the movies. We had blinders on.*

The first day was the worst. She had just sat next to Robert, in her hospital gown, slumped in a wheelchair, and wept for the baby she could not hold or nurse or comfort. Questions screamed inside her head: What did we do to deserve this? What did *I* do to cause this? How had a problem-free pregnancy—she hadn't even had any morning sickness—turned into a life-and-death struggle? One minute she's calling her doctor about a urinary tract infection because she keeps having to pee all the time, and the next minute he's telling her, *Dear, that's no infection, that's your water breaking. You've got to get to the hospital. Now.* That's how quick everything went to hell, and not even ten days in the hospital, parked in bed with an IV plugged into her arm to halt the contractions, could prepare her for the shock of seeing her Elias splayed out in the NICU like a laboratory experiment, his face so battered by the delivery that he appeared to have five o'clock shadow.

The image of him lying there would always be fixed in her memory. Because of all the bruising from the delivery, he needed extensive treatment for jaundice. The blood in his contusions, as it broke down, formed the waste product bilirubin, which in large amounts is toxic, turning the eyes and skin a jaundiced yellow. The liver cleanses the system of bilirubin, but a preemie's liver isn't very efficient to begin with, even without all the bruising. To battle this, they gave Elias phototherapy—he was lying under the bright purple-white glare of the bili lights, which helps the body break down bilirubin and get rid of it. But to Amalia, those healing rays were a merciless spotlight on every scratch, bruise, mark and imperfection. Elias's eyes were covered with gauze to protect them from the harsh UV glare—"snow goggles," Robert called them—but Amalia couldn't bring herself to smile. She had never imagined her baby could look like this.

But Patty had doused the bili lights and taken off the eye patches during that first visit so Amalia and Robert could see his face better; the nurses know how important early bonding, however tenuous, can be. That had been a little better, but still hard.

"Maybe he'll open his eyes for you," Robert had said to Amalia. Then he turned to the nurse: "She's never seen his eyes before. I have, but she didn't get the chance."

Amalia had winced a little at this comment but said nothing. Elias's eyes had stayed tightly closed. Then he had tried to cry, a silent scream stifled by the tube down his throat. Amalia had looked crushed.

"He knows your voice," Patty had suggested. "So talk to him."

And so they had, in what would become a daily ritual. At the sound of those familiar voices, his cries would slow, then stop. They had made their first connection with their new son.

That small sign, that little bond, made all the difference, turning despair into hope, even confidence. They told him all about the exciting and tense days leading up to his birth. They read from Amalia's journal. They read from a memory book left by one of the night-shift nurses, a friend of Amalia's. She had turned to a passage in which someone recalled seeing her newborn nephew for the first time: "You instantly fall in love. I thought he was the most beautiful baby in the world." Amalia read that, then turned to Robert and said, "And yes, he *is* the most beautiful baby in the world. Don't you feel that?"

He nodded. "Of course he is." But Robert's voice shook a little.

In surprisingly few days, coming to the NICU became easier. They experienced the same shift in perspective that causes neonatal nurses to view preemies as normal and full-term babies as enormous and overweight. To the Allmans, who had no other children, Elias looked, well, like a baby was supposed to look. Robert called him his "little chicken in the incubator" and delighted in combing his surprisingly full head of hair. For Thanksgiving, Amalia brought him a plant and a toy glow-worm with a face that lit up and played music. It helped that they had discovered a few things that made life easier for them: First, they came to believe that they were in very good hands, that the humanity behind the technology of the NICU was gentle, kind and patient—a place in which Elias was safe and they felt secure. Second, they saw they were far from alone: with one out of every ten American babies being born premature, Elias had plenty of company. The unit was filled with babies, many of whom had started just as shakily as Elias but who were now far along, nearing discharge. It was a comfort to see this, a graphic demonstration that the scary environment of Room 288 would eventually give way to a more "normal" one. Through the windows of the less intensive rooms, they could see moms were holding and nursing their babies, giving them baths, dressing them. Amalia felt a painful longing when she saw the attention that she could not give Elias as long as he was tied to his ventilator, but she also felt certain they would get there.

And finally, the Allmans realized they did not have to view Elias's projected three-month stay in the hospital as an unbearably long postponement of their life together as a family. Instead, the nurses framed it this way: They had not lost any time together at all; if all went well, Elias would be home by his original due date. "You weren't planning on having him before then, anyway, right?" Patty Rulon asked.

This simple, commonsense question put Elias's prematurity in a new perspective. It was the hardest lesson to accept, far tougher than comprehending the impenetrable diagram of a PDA someone handed her and all too easy to forget on days when things went badly. But they made a concerted effort to stop seeing the empty crib and the other baby things they had piled in one corner of their apartment, a nursery in the making short-circuited by Elias's premature arrival. They tried to forget about the baby announcements and cute pajamas that wouldn't fit for months: Those things would come, in their proper time.

Soon it was hard to imagine any other existence. Amalia would go to work, get off early, come to the hospital, visit for a couple hours, go home to throw some dinner together for her and Robert (mostly take-out or frozen dinners until he finally begged her to make something fresh), then the two of them would come back for the evening, sitting down in front of the incubator as if it were a television.

After those first terrible few days, things even seemed to get easy for a time. Elias seemed so clearly healthier than many of the other babies in Room 288. Not that they took comfort in others' misfortune. It was just a simple fact that, as preemies went, Elias was pretty well off, his initial progress encouraging—perhaps too encouraging. His beginning course of treatment included transfusions, antibiotics, steroids for his lungs, three courses of Indocin to close his PDA—which snapped shut just before they were about to call in the heart surgeon to discuss a possible ligation. The powerful drug shut down his kidneys as well—a normal reaction, the staff explained, but a potentially harmful one. It was corrected by a course of dopamine, a potent neurotransmitter that is useful for restoring renal function. Amalia had never realized a wet diaper could make her so happy. In celebration, the nurse let her change it—the first time. She immediately called Robert at work. "He's peeing just fine, now, honey," she declared with a smile, sounding like the parent of a kid who had just aced the SAT. "And I changed it!"

Robert, who only a few months ago had groused about not wanting to change diapers, was jealous. "I want the next one!" he crowed.

Amalia even got to watch Elias's second surfactant treatment, one of the more unusual procedures in the NICU. While his nurse gently cradled Elias inside his incubator, the respiratory therapist cranked up the ventilator to a higher pressure and concentration of oxygen, then poured into the infant's breathing tube a small vial of milky white liquid: the natural lubricant surfactant, extracted and purified from the lungs of calves. Then they slowly rotated, flipped and turned the baby in order to spread the liquid evenly and thoroughly inside his lungs, trying not to jostle the child too much or tangle the monitor leads, IV lines and respirator tubes. It was a curious sight, precise and almost ritualistic. "Like mixing a martini," one nurse joked. "Except this one's stirred, not shaken."

Elias made steady progress after that, reaching the landmark of room air on his ventilator settings by his third day of life, a fairly quick recovery given that he had needed 70 percent oxygen on his first day of life, about three times the content of normal room air. The next step would be to extubate. His eyes, lungs and mental development would all benefit from a short stay on the ventilator. Not only that, but when he came off the ventilator Amalia would be able to hold him. It was an exciting time for the Allmans; they could see, each day, the progress he made, the fading bruises, the removal of the bili lights, the removal of one drug after another from his IV tree.

But then, in the second week, his inability to feed, the gradual distention of his stomach, and his failure to move his bowels became prominent dilemmas in the daily progress notes in his chart. In a place where dirty diapers are counted and weighed and even celebrated because they are one sure measure of health, this was not a good development.

Amalia could see that Elias had begun to look worse: thinner, paler, more dependent on the ventilator. Instead of the extubation everyone had expected after he reached room air, Elias's oxygen settings began to creep back up again—30 percent, 40 percent, 45 percent—delivered at ever-greater pressures and rates. More cultures were taken in search of possible infections, more blood samples, more tests: ultrasounds, a benevolent magic wand that Amalia didn't mind, and X rays, which she hated, wincing whenever that awful buzzing machine was lowered over

Elias like some monstrous appendage, followed by the jarring call "Shooting!" The IVs began to proliferate again as Elias's delicate preemie metabolism slipped out of balance: low pH, poor electrolytes, low red cell count, high sodium. The neonatologists found themselves constantly trying to readjust his medications, but fixing one imbalance in a sick preemie often triggers another.

Meanwhile, his belly just kept getting bigger, with nothing to show for it—nothing going in, nothing going out. It was at that point that Lupe called for the surgeon.

Amalia waits anxiously for the surgeon to arrive. The fears she felt that first day in the NICU are resurfacing with full force.

One of the other nurses, Chris Merlo, who has taken over Elias's care this afternoon, is laying out the implements for the procedure: plastic tubing, a syringe, warm sterile water, plenty of towels, something called a Red Robinson, which looks like a large turkey baster. As she works, Chris tries to calm the nervous mother by telling her about the surgeon, Visut Kanchanapoom. He's something of a hospital legend, she says, a regular in the unit as long as there has been an NICU at Long Beach. The nurses adore him. He always comes in when he's needed without complaint, no matter the time, no matter the day, which is rare among prominent surgeons. Dr. Kanchanapoom is gentle and soothing with the babies and patient with the parents, and he uses special care to create the smallest possible scar. There is a procedure called a "cut-down" that is sometimes used in the NICU, a method of implanting a permanent IV catheter in babies who are going to need long-term care—a safer, more durable method of administering drugs than conventional IV needles. These cut-downs sometimes leave enormous scars on the neck or chest that are carried throughout life; Kanchanapoom's cut-downs leave an almost invisible notch, his trademark. "I take my children to Visut," Chris Merlo assures Amalia with conviction in her voice. "He is the best."

Of course, she leaves out the diminutive surgeon's more unusual qualities, his penchant for telling ribald jokes during surgery for one. And his passion for certain unproven methods of halting the aging process: human growth hormone and special drinking water from a mountainous area in the Russian state of Georgia, where the average life span is well over one hundred years. He swears by the health benefits of this personal regimen. None of this has the slightest relevance to his surgical abilities or the calm touch he reserves for the infants he treats or the fact that he is known for excelling at abdominal surgery and the correction of conditions such as gastroschisis. Kanchanapoom is a very colorful character, odd and endearing, a small man with the perfect, tapered fingers of a violinist, whose eccentricities are accepted without question because of his talent and genuine niceness in a profession where the two qualities don't always accompany each other. Lupe tells her residents that she once considered surgery as a specialty when she served her residency. "But then I looked at the talent Visut has in those hands of his, and I came to my senses—I just knew I could never do what he does."

No one seems to know exactly how old Dr. Kanchanapoom is, which is one reason not everyone dismisses out of hand his theories about aging, and why some members of the hospital staff have even adopted his regimen. There are pictures of him in 1975 in the NICU scrapbooks, smiling over a baby long since grown up. A quarter century later, every person in those pictures has aged and changed in very clear ways—except Visut Kanchanapoom. He looks the same. The surgeon just nods and smiles modestly at such observations, with Lupe providing her usual irreverent caveat: "He may look the same as he did in 1975, but you have to remember, he's always looked fifty years old, even when he was thirty."

After the three o'clock shift change, the surgeon arrives and explains to Amalia what he plans to do. He has checked the X rays and seen no evidence of a problem that would require abdominal surgery. He examines the baby, feeling his stomach, listening to the sounds emanating from his bowels, nodding and murmuring to Elias, whom he refers to as Elijah. No one corrects him. Then he goes to work.

Chris flips Elias onto his belly and holds him still as Visut inserts a thin tube into the baby's behind, gently, slowly, trying to spare the baby discomfort, though it is clear it is a losing battle. Elias writhes, his arms flailing weakly, as the surgeon begins to squirt some saline solution into the tube with the turkey baster device. Elias mouths that awful, silent cry around his breathing tube, and Amalia has to turn away. All the while, Visut softly murmurs to Elias, "Hi, baby, I know, baby, it's okay, baby." It's almost a chant, soothing and calm. Even so, Elias is clearly upset. His sats plummet, and Chris leans over to crank up the oxygen. Amalia cringes but forces herself to look directly at Elias again, almost wishing she had decided not to stay.

After about thirty seconds of flushing, some small, hard balls of matter, almost greenish in color, are washed out onto a white surgical cloth—plugs of meconium, the size of bunny pellets. The surgeon continues squirting and flushing, looking for more, but only clear water comes out. He relieves the air pressure that has built up inside Elias's intestines from the turkey baster, and Elias abruptly stops crying, as if he suddenly feels better.

Dr. Kanchanapoom looks vaguely displeased as he takes off his gloves. Chris dries and diapers Elias, settling him back down. That could have done the trick, the surgeon muses to himself, but what came out of Elias did not seem to be enough to cause a major blockage. Amalia, however, is delighted. To her, it appears the problem has been solved.

"What happens next?" she asks.

"We wait a few days," the surgeon says. "That may have eliminated the blockage. We'll have to wait and see."

21

Wʜᴇɴ Jᴜʟɪᴇ Fʀᴀɴᴄᴇ ʀᴇᴛᴜʀɴs ᴛᴏ ʜᴇʀ ᴏғғɪᴄᴇ, sʜᴇ ɢʟᴜᴍʟʏ ʟᴏᴏᴋs over her roster of nurses. A resident and a nurse are available to transport the Down Syndrome baby with the heart defect, but Julie has no one left to fetch the drug baby. She looks at the barely legible note Art Strauss scrawled: "A one-day-old suffering drug withdrawal in Cerritos, noncritical, mother and baby both tested positive for heroin and cocaine."

Memorial is one of a handful of hospitals in the region capable of bringing a baby through drug withdrawal—not to mention treating the other possible complications, from birth defects and developmental delays to the increased risk of AIDS if the mother was an IV drug user. Julie's concern is not treating the baby—it's staffing. "I don't suppose we could just say no?" she asks Art.

The medical director grins and shakes his head. Staff shortages are never a reason to turn down a patient as long as there is an open bed, he reminds her. Hospital policy.

"But I have no one to send," she complains. "Everyone is already stretched too thin."

In the end Julie decides to take the transport call herself, unusual for the coordinator. But there is simply no one else she can spare. This transport should be quick and fairly easy; Cerritos is just one town over from Long Beach in the sprawl of smaller cities south of Los Angeles. Some transports are emergencies, hair-raising rescues of children with deadly conditions, usually handled by a nurse, a respiratory therapist and a neonatal fellow or resident. This is a noncritical transport. The baby isn't on oxygen, so an RT isn't necessary, and the child is stable, with no life-threatening conditions, which means a doctor need not go, either. The dirty work of filling the holes on the next shift is done. Julie doesn't have to do her end-of-shift report to the next coordinator for two hours. She figures she can be back in an hour, maybe ninety minutes at most, traffic willing. "I need some air anyway," she says and takes off, pushing an empty transport incubator in front of her.

The ambulance fights its way through a jammed freeway to the community hospital. It's a grim, one-story brick building in a notch of Southern California seemingly untouched by the rampant prosperity fueling most of the region's economy. The maternity wing is small, the nursery mostly empty. A single nurse is on duty, greeting Julie like visiting royalty as she pushes the transport incubator in, a mobile medical kit slung over her shoulder like an unwieldy purse.

"Here's the poor thing," the nurse says, taking Julie into a side room where a small baby is crying irritably, more like a squawking bird with a wheeze than a child. The cries are interspersed with sneezes. The baby's nose is running, and she is waving her fists in a jerky, unnatural motion, almost as if she were receiving small electrical shocks. She is, in short, a miniature junkie suffering from withdrawal. The symptoms tell Julie that this child is much worse off than she had been led to believe.

"We knew what was coming as soon as we took one look at the mother," the other nurse says. "She had track marks all over her. She just showed up at the last minute. We didn't even have time to get a doctor—a nurse had to deliver the baby. She's only two hours old."

Julie shakes her head: just two hours, and already in withdrawal. Mild cases of drug abuse in pregnant women don't usually lead to withdrawal in their babies for the better part of a day. For it to kick in this fast means the mother is a major addict—and the baby is going to have a very hard time.

Julie begins to examine the infant, checking her heart and lungs while questioning the other nurse expertly, prodding her less experienced colleague to reveal what's been done so far with the baby, which isn't much: No blood tests, except for HIV, which isn't back yet. No shots. No antibiotics. No feeding. No CBC or cultures, none of the things that would have been done routinely, immediately, back at the NICU. Like many hospitals, this one simply is not set up for sick babies.

"We didn't want to do much," the nurse explains. "You guys are the experts." As she speaks, she's looking over Julie's shoulder at the baby as the NICU nurse flips the child and removes her diaper. The other nurse says, "Oooh, that's a bad rash."

The baby's bottom is red and almost excoriated, as if burned by acid. "It's from the drugs," Julie explains. "Their feces become very acidic. God, this kid's a mess."

The girl is a classic drug baby. She's wasted, with almost no body fat, almost as if she were a preemie or a concentration camp survivor, even though she is close to full term. She has been throwing up, unable to keep much formula down, probably dehydrated, her blood sugar and electrolytes out of whack. She is way beyond cranky, inconsolable, unable to calm down, unable to sleep more than a few minutes at a time. Her expression is not that of a healthy crying infant—the screwed-up, red-faced, pick-me-up expression—but a hollow-cheeked, twitching look of pain for which there is little relief beyond time and a steady diet of morphine, gradually weaned over the course of days or weeks. There is no such thing as cold turkey in the NICU, where drug withdrawal is a life-threatening condition.

"Mom said she had given up the drugs but just started in the last couple of weeks," the nurse tells Julie.

"That's a lie," Julie mutters, not looking up from the baby, who promptly vomits all over the clean clothes she has just put on her. Julie starts dressing her again. In the late eighties and early nineties, Julie became an expert on drug babies, mostly children of crack addicts. With the crack epidemic largely over, the numbers have declined, though there are still always several drug babies in the NICU as heroin has made a bit of a comeback. Back then, the unit was filled with cocaine-exposed preemies—at times it seemed it was every other baby. She knows from bitter experience that it takes months, not weeks, of drug abuse to produce a child like this one—and that addicts usually under-report their abuse, even if it means keeping important information from the doctors and nurses treating the baby.

It was once feared that such children would never be able to bond, that drug abusers were creating an army of psychopaths, born to pain, unable to forge relationships, forever angry and alone. Those fears turned out to be overblown; patience, treatment, love and kindness can do a lot for these kids over time. It was hard at first, and for a long time the babies behaved as if being held and talked to and loved were painful, even intolerable experiences. But they eventually did okay, Julie found—most of them, anyway. "We're gonna take care of you," Julie tells the girl, who wails even louder, the gentle touch and voice causing her real pain, so raw is her abused nervous system. "I know, honey, I know. It hurts."

Julie wraps the baby in a receiving blanket very tightly, leaving her no room to move. Drug babies often respond well to this "baby bur-rito" treatment; the straitjacket bundling seems to comfort them. The little girl's cries do indeed slow, and she seems to relax. Back at the unit, there are automated cribs that rock babies rhythmically for hours on end. Sometimes this is the only way to soothe infants who are born ad-dicted. The other nurse says, "Mom has two other kids, eleven, twelve years old. They were both taken from her, given to the grandmother."

Julie nods. It's a familiar cycle, moms with drug babies having one after another. Just a month ago, they treated a drug baby infected with AIDS. Her mother had given birth to another infant a year earlier, also HIV-positive, now dead. The father, an HIV carrier as well, was on a mission to impregnate as many young women as possible before he died. The case was a nightmare.

"Mom is thirty-one," the other nurse continues. "She looks fifty-one, though. Maybe more."

As these words are uttered, the baby's mother hobbles into the room just in time to hear the observation. She doesn't react to it, though. Julie glances at her and figures every look in the mirror tells this woman that fifty-one is a generous estimate. She is small and stooped, her hair a wild, dirty gray mane. She is wearing a faded white-and-paisley hospital gown and a flannel robe, her arms protruding from the short sleeves in all their scabrous junkie glory. She sits down heavily and looks fearfully at Julie as a medical technician, who followed her into the room, wraps a tourniquet around her left arm and jabs her with a needle to draw a blood sample. The woman howls and stamps her feet in pain without ever looking at the tech or her arm. She has a peculiar, disconnected look.

In a slow, careful voice, Julie tells the woman who she is and why she is here. The woman nods. She seems to accept as a given that babies must be taken from mothers for their own good, as if that were the norm. Julie is patient with her, her voice neutral, betraying none of the anger she feels for this woman. She prides herself on her professionalism. She also needs this woman's cooperation.

"Your baby is extremely irritable now and showing other signs of withdrawal from the drugs you took during your pregnancy. That's why she looks and acts like this." Julie is holding the baby now, gently rocking her.

The woman just stares, then howls again as the tech, unable to get blood from her ruined arteries, sticks her again for another try. Julie continues, "I need to ask you some questions. Was it cocaine and heroin?"

The woman looks at her blankly. The tech sticks her a third time, and she stamps her feet again, stifling her yells behind gritted, yellow teeth. Two of her front teeth are missing.

"I need to know," Julie says. "It will help us treat the baby. Was it cocaine or heroin or both?"

Reluctantly, the woman nods. "Both. But only for the last four weeks."

Julie arches an eyebrow and the woman looks down at her feet, but she sticks to her story: "I was clean, except for the last four weeks." She says this as if she feels she deserves credit for the accomplishment.

The tech, who has been squatting next to the woman, stands up in disgust. "I can't get anything out of her. I'm going to get Bobby. He can get blood out of a stone." He walks out.

"Told ya," the mother says, smiling faintly. "You can't get anything out of these arms."

Julie hands the woman some papers to sign, authorizing the baby's transport to Long Beach, authorizing treatments, IV lines, drug therapies. It is one of medicine's ironies that the woman who caused this child's illness is also the only person who can authorize treatment, at least until the courts get involved, which takes a while. As the woman accepts the papers and pen in shaking hands, Julie explains where the NICU is located, how treatment for the baby's drug addiction will begin immediately, and how the unit's liberal visiting policies allow parents to be with their babies around the clock.

The woman seems surprised at this. "I can visit?"

"Oh yes, absolutely," Julie says. "We encourage you to visit and participate in the care of your baby." She hands her a card with the unit's address and phone number. "What's the baby's name?"

"Ella," the mother says. "I mean Elena. No, I mean Ella."

Julie looks at her. The woman is apparently deciding what to name her girl as they speak. "Ella," she says with finality, and Julie writes it down.

"We're going to give her morphine to ease her withdrawal, then gradually wean her from that. It'll take a while."

Outside in the hallway, peering into the nursery through glass windows, are three women and two children, all of them crying. "My mom, my sisters and my other kids," the woman says miserably. "They're upset that you have to take the baby."

"What about the father?" Julie asks.

"Oh, he's not coming. He's too scared. He's not . . . from here."

Julie realizes the woman is afraid that the hospital will call the immigration authorities. "Listen, we don't call anyone. We have other things to worry about."

"Well," the mom says, "he doesn't get off from work until eight."

Julie looks up from her paperwork. "I just need his name for the records."

The woman sighs. "Just put down 'Unknown.'"

Julie runs through the questions on her admission form. Insurance, no. Prenatal care, no. Family physician, none. Cigarette smoking, yes, about forty cigarettes a day. Julie flinches at this. Forty cigarettes a day while pregnant provides toxic doses of nicotine to the fetus and radically diminishes the unborn child's oxygen supply. The damage from the smoking, she knows, could be even worse than the damage from the drugs. Statistically, such babies are more likely to have developmental delays and other problems in later life.

Another technician, Bobby, proves his reputation is deserved by walking in, jabbing the mom, and getting blood on the first draw. Julie is horrified to see that he is not wearing gloves. He blots the woman's bleeding arm and holds the cotton in his bare hand. In this age of AIDS, such casual handling of blood and sharps—with an IV drug user, no less—is an incredible gaffe and incredibly dangerous. No one else seems to notice, however, and Julie just shakes her head, anxious to wrap things up and just get out of there.

"Can't I just take my baby home?" the mother whimpers.

Julie can barely contain herself at this. The county social worker has already been in and signed an emergency removal order. The mother knows this. And the baby is clearly sick. She's twisting in Julie's arms, constantly in motion, trying to suck her fingers, trying to comfort herself, trying to cope with the fact that her insides are on fire. It breaks Julie's heart. Her NICU is filled with parents who did everything right for their babies, who watched every calorie, took every test, gave up every bad habit—and who still have to cope with babies born profoundly ill, through no one's fault but nature's. They would give anything for a shot at a normal kid like Ella, whose sickness is, as far as Julie is concerned, a product of a mother's selfishness. And nothing will be done. The government will pick up the tab for both the mother's and child's care. There will be no legal consequences. This is the mother's third child to be exposed to drugs and raised by the state. Julie suppresses her anger but does not mince words.

"Ella cannot go home with you or anyone else. She has to be hospitalized and treated. Even if social services were not involved, she could not go home with you. She's sick, and she's acting this way because of the drugs you took."

The woman begins to sniffle, and a few tears run down her wrinkled, pallid cheeks. "I know," she says. Then she turns to the other nurse and asks, with unabashed eagerness, "Do you think I can get something? For the pain, I mean? Like my baby is going to get?"

A short time later, Ella is safely stowed in the transport incubator, still wailing, with Julie sitting next to her for the ride home. "What kind of life are you going to have, pumpkin?" she asks the child, shaking her head. "Think they can find you a better mom?"

Back at the unit, she weighs Ella, measures her, puts salve on her wounded behind and changes her. Then she scores Ella on a scale that measures her degree of drug withdrawal, based upon behavior, symptoms, heart rate and other indicators. The scale is one to twenty, with twenty being the worst and one being no withdrawal symptoms at all.

Ella scores a twenty.

"It's pretty bad," Julie tells Art as she returns to her office.

"Well, let's get Sara Masur involved. If anyone can calm her down, she can."

Julie nods, but she's already on the run. It's time to give her report to the swing-shift coordinator. And the secretary is waving the telephone at her and saying, "You're not going to like this. There's another transport." Meanwhile, Lupe Padilla is in the coordinator's office on another phone line, sounding agitated and giving Julie looks as if to say another problem is about to land in her lap. Lupe rolls her eyes and mouths a word Julie did not want to hear: "Twins." And then: "Twenty-seven-weekers. Bad."

22

NOT EVERY BABY WHO ARRIVES IN THE NICU IS IN CRITICAL condition or in need of a ventilator or multiple IVs or resuscitation. Many are not sick at all—the rule-out sepsis babies, who stay for only three days then go home, or kids with bad cases of jaundice, who need some phototherapy but are otherwise fine. Even those with infections detected early can be in and out in a week or ten days, never even seeming ill except for a fever and crankiness, needing nothing more than a course of antibiotics. And then there are babies who require little in the way of dramatic, immediate treatment, though their problems are severe, even devastating to their families. Little Jordan Leos, the other infant transported to the NICU today, is one such child.

He is two days old, limp and pale, with wispy black curls and very small at just over four pounds. His cry is weak. He is one month premature, small for his gestational age (SGA, another NICU acronym for his chart) and showing signs of infection and mild respiratory difficulty. He arrived via ambulance early in the afternoon, with his anxious parents, sister and brother trailing behind in their car, his mother calm and concerned, his father shaky, almost in shock.

Still, Jordan is breathing on his own and needs no ventilator, though he is receiving oxygen through a nasal canula, a two-pronged hose that fits in his nose. Because he is in no immediate danger and space is at a premium, he was initially put in the less intensive Room

276. Some of the babies in here are on ventilators, some just oxygen, some on room air but too sick for less intensive settings.

Jordan's principal diagnosis is Down Syndrome, something his family learned of through prenatal testing very early in the pregnancy. With two perfectly healthy kids, eight and six years old, and no problems with their births, it was stunning to sit down with their doctor one day and hear that a misfired split of chromosomes had been detected in their unborn child

"You get the results of that test, and your whole life changes in a split second," Maricela Leos tells Dr. Jose Perez as she gazes at her son. "It takes a minute to sink in, you know? But then you say, 'Okay. Now what?' They wanted to know if we wanted to discuss terminating the pregnancy, but we never really considered it. We knew things would be harder for him but not insurmountable. Maybe a little special. Maybe needing a little more care. But not all that different."

Jose is nodding. He likes this mom, pleased at the obvious thought she has given her son and his future—and by her willingness to embrace a less-than-perfect child whose future is very much an unknown. There is a strength about her, a bedrock belief that things will turn out okay. Just one day after his birth, she seems grounded and ready for this challenge, which is not often the case in the stressful confines of the NICU, where going to pieces is the norm.

It helps that Mr. and Mrs. Leos know this isn't their fault. Nothing they did caused Jordan to have three twenty-first chromosomes instead of two, and there is nothing they could have done to stop it. This is a random genetic flaw, one that happens in the egg or sperm cell before conception once in every thousand or so births, making it one of the most common genetic problems. The cause is unknown, though DNA research holds out hope that someday the condition will be reversible. For now, nothing can be done about the chain of events inside the womb. The developing embryo is stuck with that extra chromosome, and every cell in the body follows the same flawed road map, replicating the extra strands of DNA over and over, leading to all the classic symptoms of Down's: the flattened facial features, small forehead, short index fingers, impaired mental development.

"What we weren't ready for was his heart," Enrique Leos adds, unable to suppress the sadness in his voice. "We knew a lot of Down Syndrome babies have heart problems, but we were hoping . . ."

He trails off. Half of all Down's babies have heart defects as well. Again, despite decades of study, no one knows why. Jordan is one of the unlucky 50 percent. He has a heart condition called tetralogy of Fallot, a package of four separate defects in the construction of the heart that, in combination, cause diminished oxygenation of the blood, one of the ailments that can cause "blue baby syndrome." It can be corrected surgically or made less severe with the installation of a shunt in the blood vessels around the heart, a sort of reverse PDA. But this is generally done when the child is several months old or even approaching his first birthday, giving him time to grow, and grow stronger. The tetralogy was diagnosed before Jordan's transport; indeed, it is the reason for it.

Jose explains that while his heart condition is not immediately life-threatening, it means Jordan will be subject to bouts of cyanosis, in which his body will be deprived of sufficient oxygen. He will turn pale, his lips will turn bluish, and he'll need more oxygen then. He will be at risk of apnea—dangerous pauses in his breathing—and will need to be monitored electronically when he sleeps, even after he goes home. He will tire easily, and the ailment, in combination with Down Syndrome, explains his small size. He may also have problems feeding. Doctors from the pediatric section of the hospital's Heart Institute will be working closely with the neonatologists on Jordan's case, he says.

"The good news is," says Jose, always the optimist, "that his heart condition does not appear to be as severe as many, which means he should do well here." The look of relief on Jordan's parents is unmistakable; they have been on the roller coaster all day.

Later, Jordan's nurse, Jody King, gently raises the subject of Down Syndrome again. She is concerned that the parents' focus has been on the baby's heart and worried about how they will react to Jordan's differentness, the developmental delays he is likely to experience, the differences in his appearance, the special classes and treatment he may need to ensure he does as well in life as possible. Some parents, devastated by their child's condition, by the stigma associated with "mental retardation," have a great deal of trouble accepting it—and their child. Some even go into a kind of mourning, as if their baby had died.

So Jody tells the Leoses about various support groups in the area for parents of Down's children, trying to be as encouraging as possible. "You know, a lot of Down's babies do quite well and function at a very high level. Like that actor on television, remember him?" Jordan's parents nod at this but say nothing, so Jody presses on: "Have you been around children with Down Syndrome before?"

Enrique smiles at this, but his voice quavers a bit: "Oh yes. I'm a school bus driver for special students. I transport them all the time. I know they can be great kids. I love them."

Jody can hear the sincerity in his voice and relaxes, turning to the baby. "Well, Jordan," she says, "I think you chose your parents well."

"What's that you're giving him?" Maricela asks, pointing to an IV.

Jody explains the breathing patterns of a baby with tetralogy of Fallot and the need to clear his lungs of fluid, which is why he is receiving diuretics through an intravenous line. This will be another constant source of trouble to look out for: the buildup of fluid in his lungs, which can be caused by the sluggish blood flow associated with his heart condition. She looks intently at the mother, whose expression is one of intense concentration as she absorbs Jody's information. "You've got a lot to learn, don't you?" the nurse asks.

"Yes, but that's good," Maricela answers immediately, never taking her eyes off her baby. "I want to learn."

Enrique, meanwhile, is leaning over his son, lost in his own thoughts. His son and daughter are on tiptoes outside in the hallway, peering in at their new brother through a window; children are allowed to visit in the NICU only on weekends, and they are losing patience at being excluded. He gives them a smile and a wink. Then he gives Jordan a gentle kiss on the forehead, right below his wispy black hair, careful not to scratch him with the rough stubble on his face—Enrique hasn't shaved, or slept, for that matter, in more than twenty-four hours.

"I hoped that the first test was wrong," Enrique Leos confesses to his son, "and that you would be okay. And then we had the amniocentesis and we found out it was for sure. And I realized, I will be driving my son on my bus with all the other special kids."

Father is lovingly stroking son's face now, a few tears spilling onto his stubbly cheeks. "Now, wouldn't that be something, huh, Jordan?"

23

It's lunchtime in the NICU break room. Decompression time.

A dozen nurses are gathered around the two long folding tables pushed together in the center of the room, picking at cafeteria trays or microwaved meals. Two others are stretched out on vinyl-covered couches, one resting, one napping for fifteen minutes, trying to make it through a double shift.

More than just a place for meals, the break room is a place to blow off steam, talk about the patients, the doctors, the hospital administration, the long hours, families, husbands, kids and boyfriends. Jokes are traded like recipes, stories about the good old days (*Remember the time we taped the door shut on the residents' call room with the resident inside, then beeped him to a Code Blue?*) are told and retold, anything to wind the stress down a notch. The nurses' lounge, more than any other part of the NICU, is the place to go to get the latest information on just about anything, from hospital policies to the lowdown on the best and worst doctors in the hospital, from which nurses are feuding with whom to which residents are liked and which ones the nurses would prefer to anesthetize and stick in a closet.

There are always four or five different conversations in progress at the table. In the background, daytime TV drones on a set bolted to the wall. Today the conversation focuses on the brutal hours, the overtime, the mandating. Julie France hides behind her soda can and asks, "You're not going to start a food fight with me, are you?"

The topic's too sensitive for anyone to laugh, but the conversational tide shifts to the patients, what a sad little dude David Rios is, whether poor Nikkol Hawkshaw will ever be able to eat, how great little Miracle is doing. And then there is Baby Girl Berger, Lupe's awful code case in the OR a few weeks earlier. The child has just returned from her lung treatments with nitric oxide at Los Angeles Children's Hospital and has surprised everyone who sees her with her dramatic recovery.

"I didn't even recognize her," says Kim Holloway, one of the NICU's most outspoken nurses, who regularly cares for the sickest babies. "We all expected a vegetable to come back, and this kid looks *good*. My own babies never looked that good."

It's true. The amazing resilience of newborns has worked in the Bergers' favor. Despite her near-death experience, despite twelve minutes at zero on the Apgar chart, she is showing far fewer signs of damage than expected. She has no seizures, she is not "posturing"—making the rigid grimaces and arm and leg flexing often seen in brain-damaged babies—and, most important, she is sucking and swallowing and feeding normally. Sara Masur couldn't believe her eyes.

To be sure, there is a note of caution in all this. The nurses have an expression, "It's easy to be a baby," which is another way of saying that the tasks infants need to master to survive do not require many higher brain functions. Tougher milestones will come later: when she tries to sit up, to crawl, to walk, to speak. But everyone agrees that she has already come a long way. Most babies who have been through similar experiences never learn to suck; they have to be tube-fed, sometimes for their whole lives, Kim says. "I have to admit, when she was delivered I wasn't sure we had done the right thing. I mean, she looked *so* bad."

"The ethics of this are so murky," Karol Norris, the unit's clinical nurse specialist, agrees. "You always wonder if you've gone too far with a code, but you can never *know* until later—like with this girl. We had another kid years ago, he was tiny on the fetal ultrasound, less than four hundred grams, and we were told the mom was only in her twenty-second, maybe twenty-third week. At the delivery the resident didn't want to do much, just let the baby go, but I called Jose. I thought the baby was older, that the ultrasound had been misleading, that the dates were off and he was just very small for his gestational age. And Jose agreed with me. We resuscitated the child, and he turned out to be a twenty-*eight*-weeker, definitely viable. Like Allman or Hachigan. He's fine now. So a lot of times we just have to go all the way and hope for the best."

They mention another patient, a kid who won't eat and is far too thin, and that talk inevitably segues into how hard it is to find a dress that fits for the NICU Christmas party, how hard it is to get rid of the ten extra pounds everyone would like to shed, how tough it is to get by on a nurse's salary, particularly for the newer nurses, who find themselves living paycheck to paycheck, with each check spent before it arrives. All the overtime seems to go to taxes, they complain. "Nowhere can you work harder and longer for less money and respect than here," Julie agrees cheerfully. "That's why we love it here."

"That would be one working definition of the word 'nurse,'" Kim agrees.

Like nurses everywhere, NICU nurses are expert complainers—it is a recreational activity for them, usually lighthearted. But sometimes it is underscored by a genuine anger, and money is often at the root of it. The subject shifts again, this time to Medicaid cheats. This is a heated topic for the nurses, several of whom do home health follow-ups on kids discharged from the NICU. During these visits, the nurses make sure their former patients are getting the care they need, and they also get the chance to maintain friendships with parents and bonds they forged with the babies in the unit. Mostly, they see families struggling to make ends meet while caring for a medically needy child. But they also see a number of families who have substantial assets—nice homes, new cars, good jobs—who have managed to qualify for a government insurance program intended for the poor, their hundred-thousand-dollar-plus hospital bills taken care of by the state rather than their own, less generous private insurance. The nurses are helpless to do anything about it because they are in the business of caring for sick kids, not policing insurance frauds. If the nurses were to get a reputation for informing on people for their insurance abuses, some parents might stop allowing the home health visits, which are essential, even lifesaving.

"We have to think of the babies and just grit our teeth," Julie tells a new nurse, who wanted to know why they don't report such abuses. "One of our nurses went to one home, and the baby was just wasting away. The mother was clueless. They couldn't figure out what was wrong. Then the nurse asks the mom to show how she was mixing the baby bottles. She was supposed to be putting one scoop of formula powder for every two ounces of water. But she was putting one scoop for a whole eight-ounce bottle. She was starving the kid! If we hadn't been welcome there, who knows what would have happened to that baby?"

The new nurse shakes her head, but the point hits home: An NICU nurse has awesome and not always easy-to-define responsibilities. They are expected to act independently, to be more than just appendages for the doctors to order about, to make treatment decisions and recommendations, which is why so many of them love the work. Nurses in other departments enjoy no such autonomy. But this independence means having to confront difficult and sometimes morally ambiguous situations, as in tolerating welfare cheats to achieve a greater good. Julie France's easy ability to explain this with a simple story or offhand remark, teaching without appearing to teach, is one of her great assets as a coordinator.

She has been here since 1986, before some of the great strides that transformed neonatal care, a young, new nurse, uncertain and fearful. The unit had just lost a number of its older nurses, and instead of languishing on the night shift for years, as happens with most newcomers, she was given a coveted day-shift slot after only five months on the job. She was inexperienced but bright and talented, and she was placed in Room 288, by far the youngest nurse in the unit's most intensive room, which was as crowded and as filled with sick babies on Julie's first day as it is today, thirteen years later.

There's a saying in hospitals, "Nurses eat their young," in recognition of the tendency of some veteran nurses to steamroller newcomers into submission. Or resignation. At the time, the toughest nurse in the place took particular delight in torturing "new meat," as she called the new nurses, testing them for weaknesses and sparing no one. You have to be tough to do this job, she'd say, justifying her manners. She'd bully new nurses into tears if she could manage it. The idea of Julie France, a nurse with just five months under her belt, working days in Room 288—the most elite assignment for a neonatal nurse—infuriated her.

On Julie's first day shift, she greeted Julie with a withering glance, looked at the baby she was assigned to care for that day—a very ill preemie—and declared flatly, loud enough for everyone to hear, "She's too new for that baby. She can't take care of him." She made a point of using the third person, as if Julie weren't standing five feet away.

Everyone in the room looked up except Julie, who just stared at the incubator in front of her, her face burning. She felt as if the school bully was about to chase her off the playground. She didn't know what to say. As the least experienced nurse on her shift, she wondered if the bully was right: What if something terrible happened to the baby because of her inexperience? The older nurse must have sensed Julie's doubts. She wore a look of triumph and announced, again very loudly, that she was going to talk to the coordinator. "I'm going to put a stop to this right now."

Then a voice came from across the room, very calm but very firm. It was Penny Jacinto, who at the time was a neonatal fellow finishing her training. Even then, Penny had no problem asserting her authority. "I want Julie to have that baby," she said with certainty. And she smiled warmly at Julie, who instantly became a fan of the young neonatologist. The bully looked astonished. She glared, hesitated, but then backed down, grumbling and red-faced with embarrassment. Julie finished the shift without a hitch, and she knew Room 288 was the place she wanted to work every day. When Julie became coordinator, she made sure new nurses were never treated as she had been. No one on Julie's watch eats the young.

"What we do here is important," she tells the new nurses. "Think about it: What do people come to a hospital for? They come for the nursing care. Your doctor isn't going to stay with you or your child all day. *We* are. We're the ones who deal with the families. *We* take their calls at three in the morning when a mom can't sleep and just has to know how her baby is doing. *We* hold their hands when their kids go to surgery. *We* snap their pictures and fuss over all those tiny newborn moments—the first time Dad holds his baby, their first bath, the last day in the hospital. *We're* the ones who have to comfort them when there are setbacks, and it's the nurses who have to clean and dress up the babies who don't make it. *We're* the ones who do it all, no one else. And that's what people come to a hospital for."

It's a good spiel, and a sincere one. Julie considers her nurses to be among the elite and their job immensely important. Privately, though, she reveals a more cynical side, acknowledging the reality that every NICU nurse must confront: responsibilities, stress and hard work that far outstrip compensation, clout and recognition. The growing sentiment that they are undervalued by their hospital has ignited some serious union organization activity for the first time in ten years, serious enough for the hospital to have hired antiunion consultants, which seems to have backfired by further spurring the feelings of disaffection. If you want to see how much the medical establishment really values nurses, Julie says, just look at your hospital bill: Every doctor's consultation, every injection, every test, every technician, every diaper and wipe and smear of A and D ointment will be itemized, charged and tallied on that bill. But nurses will not be mentioned anywhere. In the world of hospital accounting, Julie France likes to say, "The nurse just comes with the bed, like any other piece of furniture in the room."

24

Of the babies who were in Room 288 on the day Elias Allman entered the world, Steven Eric Hachigan is the first to graduate to a less intensive room—or at least the first to do it without a quick and disappointing return, as Eric Lee and Nikkol Hawkshaw did.

Like Elias, Steven was born at twenty-eight weeks. But unlike other babies in the room, only traditional preemie respiratory problems held him back. He never had an infection, never had gut problems, never had bleeding in his brain, though he was at risk for all these things. He is the basic preemie, the sort of baby whose survival would have been impossible in the sixties, before ventilators were available, dicey in the early seventies, when ventilator technology was so primitive the settings had to be made with a stopwatch instead of the computer readouts now in place, and difficult in the eighties—without surfactant, his time on the ventilator could have been many months instead of three weeks.

Monique Hachigan arrives in the unit this morning nervous with anticipation. She was told the day before Steven might be extubated, that his settings had been turned down very low with no ill effects, the last step before removing the machine entirely. But there had been false alarms in the past, when he hadn't been quite ready, and she had deliberately suppressed her hopes, fearing another disappointment. Monique Hachigan is a smart and caring woman, but a sheltered one.

She has a fragile, porcelain beauty that at times seems a reflection of her personality; her fears for her baby, amplified by having had a far healthier, older preemie, are not easily held at bay.

But there he is, in Room 276, the bulky respirator hose gone, the ET tube down his throat gone, the hiss and click and rattle of that damn ventilator gone. Gone, too, is the "mustache," a piece of white surgical tape pasted over Steven's upper lip, to which his breathing tube was sutured to hold it in place. Since his birth, all the apparatus and attachments kept her baby's face hidden from view. Now she can see him clearly for the first time. He has the wrinkled face of an old man, thin, long and pale; he's borderline anemic from all the blood drawn from him, which his tiny body cannot replace fast enough. He'll be getting a transfusion later, which should help his color and his strength, but Monique doesn't care. To her, he is a beautiful sight, a wonder. Her hands fly to her face, and she whispers, "It's a miracle. I can see him."

Margie Perez, Steven's nurse, says, "Looks great, doesn't he?"

Monique nods, her eyes welling.

"Want to hold him?" Margie asks with a smile, reaching into the incubator.

The first time a mother holds her baby in the NICU is a landmark. Denied that ritual at birth because of his respiratory distress, denied that closeness because of his ventilator and fragile health, Monique has waited patiently for the day to come. She had thought she would be prepared for the experience of having Steven in the NICU because of Paul's prematurity three years earlier. I know the drill, she had told herself. I can handle it. But the enormous gulf between a twenty-eight-weeker and a thirty-two-weeker was immediately, painfully apparent.

Paul had been big and hearty, his stay in the NICU brief compared to Steven's, a matter of weeks. His worst lingering health problem may be a lazy eye, nothing that can't be fixed. But Steven faces all sorts of potential health problems. He seems to sleep all the time, rousing only to protest with a silent, stifled cry when someone comes to take a blood sample. Watching him over the past month, seeing his painful struggle to breathe, to eat, to withstand the endless needle sticks and IV punctures, Monique has come to question everything about herself.

She has berated herself for taking Paul out costume shopping and to a Halloween party the afternoon she went into premature labor, as if that somehow caused her son's prematurity—notwithstanding the fact she had been sitting throughout the party, and was doing nothing more vigorous than stirring a pot of soup when the contractions started in earnest. She questioned the wisdom of the fertility treatments she endured to get pregnant with Steven. Maybe, she thought in her darkest moments, Steven's illness was evidence that she had not been meant to have more children. Self-doubt is normal in the NICU, and the more a parent cares, the more deeply they cut. The only cure for them is seeing progress. Monique Hachigan has waited a long month to see even one small sign that her son is getting better.

Now she sits down in one of the unit's battered orange vinyl and chrome chairs, and Margie hands her the bundled baby. Monitor wires poke out of Steven's blanket and lead back to the incubator. He is still receiving oxygen through a nasal canula, a thin plastic hose that trails behind him like a transparent tail, because his dreadful habit of forgetting to breathe—apnea—continues. But Monique seems oblivious to anything but that face staring up at her, his blue-gray newborn eyes open for a change. Sitting here with her child in her arms, warm, nestled, all her fears seem to slip away. All the doubts that have eaten at her for the last month seem to fade in importance. She knows her son has a long way to go. He has to learn to eat, he has to learn to breathe right, he has to make it through the night without setting off alarms. But she also knows, for the first time, that he is going to make it. It's no longer hope. She *knows*.

Weaning from the ventilator is a gradual process, painfully slow out of necessity. There is no such thing as going cold turkey from the vent. It was a long, halting march to get Steven Hachigan down to room air and using his lungs on his own.

But the next stage of development in the NICU, feeding, is a different story. When it happens, when a baby like Steven Hachigan turns the next corner, the neonatologists have a saying to describe it: "The switch just went on." It is that abrupt, like a lightbulb coming on. One day, a baby will need to be hand-bagged every time he gets upset or tries a bottle; the next, he cries and sucks lustily, without an errant blip on the heart monitor. With Steven, the switch went on when he was in Sara Masur's arms.

The unit's occupational therapist had been called to see him a week or so after he was extubated. The nurses had reported that he was having feeding problems: He was not making progress toward the next big milestone. His digestion was fine. There were none of the stomach or intestinal problems plaguing some of the other babies. All his nourishment was by mouth, with no more IV lines going into him, which meant his chances of getting an infection of some sort had gone from fairly high to virtually zero. The lifegiving intravenous lines, necessary as they are, are best pulled out as soon as possible in order to shut off that pathway into the body for bacteria, virus and other pathogens.

But most of his food was going in through the gavage tube, the force-feeding of formula and breast milk right into his stomach. He balked at "nippling," as it is called when babies learn to take a bottle or breast directly. He choked, desatted and basically turned blue whenever it was tried, managing less than an ounce of formula at a time, far too little for a single feeding. The nurses began to say he had a "feeding aversion."

"Sure, he has a feeding aversion," Sara agreed when she reviewed Steven's chart. "Because we inadvertently *taught* him to have one."

She removes the baby from his incubator. He stiffens at the strange touch, then releases some of the tension as Sara rocks him gently, not rushing to grab the bottle but taking her time, making him comfortable. His oxygen saturation, which had started to dip, eases back up again, the number on the monitor ticking back up from 83 to 89 to 97, where it belongs.

"It's not that there's anything wrong with him," Sara continues. "He's reacting in a very predictable way to what we've done to him here. And until we change that, he's going to continue to resist nippling."

She talks to him gently, brushes back his blond hair, feeling the areas of his body that are stiff and need to relax before he is ready. As usual when Sara holds a baby, she conveys the impression that there is nowhere else she needs to be, nowhere better she wants to go—though in fact her schedule is murderous. With her long brown hair in a pile on top of her head, her youthful features and her street clothes, she could easily be mistaken for one of the young mothers. Her touch is loving, soothing. Steven closes his eyes, but she gently says, "No, let's wake up now, sleepyhead. Time to go to work."

Sara Masur made her career choice by age fifteen, when a family in her Cincinnati neighborhood invited her to accompany their disabled son to therapy. She had already been his baby-sitter and readily agreed to the new duty, soon making it a regular part of her week. Each time they went, she could see his progress in overcoming his sensory problems—his brain, probably because of an injury at or before birth, had trouble processing the information his eyes and ears took in. Things got jumbled for him. Sara saw a whole new world open up for her as she watched the puzzle pieces slowly unscramble for this boy. Sara had found what she wanted to do with her life.

She had already proven—to herself and her family, at least—that she had a natural intuition that could be quite extraordinary. She could sense when others were troubled or in pain. Throughout her childhood, she would have premonitions that invariably seemed to come true: an illness in the family, the death of her grandmother. This is not anything she attempts to explain or advertise. But it is part of her unique approach to her work, something not contained in the occupational therapy texts she studied in college or the thick manuals on the shelves of her modest office; closer, perhaps, to some of the more unusual studies she has undertaken over the years, from the healing traditions of certain Native American tribes to controversial theories about the craniosacral system—the fluids and membranes that surround and protect the brain and spinal cord. Using a touch as light as the weight of a nickel on the skin, Sara attempts to sense where a child needs therapeutic massage or a gentle flexing or a warming touch. No X ray or ultrasound can reveal the soft-tissue and nerve-ending traumas Sara works on; she must find them on her own, in her own way, helping infants overcome the terrors of intubation, ventilation, the unnatural and stiff postures the NICU inflicts on them.

By traditional definition, an occupational therapist works with a person's fine motor skills (as opposed to a physical therapist, who concentrates on large motor skills). But Sara's work goes far beyond that. She is most concerned with infant development, which became a major concern in neonatology only in the last decade of the millennium. Recent studies have shown that premature babies tend to lag behind full-term children when they reach school, long after their medical conditions have been resolved. This is not true of all premature babies, but on average, it seems that something about prematurity—or something about care in the NICU—is impairing their mental, emotional and physical growth. Sara's goal is to help close that gap, to help the infants cope with and move beyond the artificial and often painful environment of the NICU and still do all the things a baby needs to do to live, grow and thrive.

The gap between the full-term and premature babies is painfully obvious in Steven Hachigan's feeding problems. In the last ten weeks of gestation, the human fetus begins to separate from the mother's biorhythms. Up until that point, the child in the womb is in time with the mother: heartbeat, sleeping, even the halting attempts to breathe with fluid-filled fetal lungs are all in step with the mother's. But at the thirty-week mark, the fetus begins to practice being awake and moving on his own time. He practices sleeping on his own time. And he practices sucking and swallowing. This is not a random pattern. There is a purpose to these exercises: sucking and swallowing and breathing may separately be instinctual behaviors, but coordinating all three is a *learned* behavior. And so when a baby is born at term, all the necessary skills for living in the outside world have already been acquired *in utero*. By the time the baby comes out, there's nothing left to learn. The practice in the womb has formed the connections in the brain that tell him how to suck, swallow and breathe without choking to death.

Preemies, however, miss out on that practice. Steven had a tube jammed down his windpipe, with a machine breathing for him when he should have been in the womb beginning these exercises. Without the experience, the practice, the connections have not been forged in Steven's brain. He is not ready. And so when the nipple is stuck in his mouth, he's not sure what to do: Should I swallow? Should I breathe? If he does the wrong thing in the wrong order, he gags or chokes or, as happens most of the time, he simply holds his breath until his oxygen saturation falls and he starts to turn blue. The nurses then take away the bottle and crank up his oxygen until he breathes again and his color comes back. He's fine. But then, when they offer the bottle again, he fights it. His brain has learned that the bottle asphyxiates him. He equates nippling with a threat to his survival.

"You're doing exactly what you've been trained to do, aren't you, Steven?" she tells the baby reassuringly. "Well, let's try something else."

Sara produces one of the special low-flow nipples she buys herself and puts it on a bottle of formula. Instead of a mouthful of milk, he will get only a few drops when he sucks. This is crucial because Steven breathes fast, not uncommon in preemies with weak lungs. With a regular nipple, he quickly gets a mouthful of milk, and before he can swallow, he has the overpowering urge to take a breath. This gives him a sensation almost like drowning, triggering his feeding problems. He doesn't want to drown, so he refuses to eat. Or he eats but doesn't breathe, which has the same effect in the end: The bottle is taken away.

Now, with the right nipple and a slow flow, this cycle can be broken. He should be able to swallow the little bit of milk that enters his mouth, rest between sucks, take a breath, and, it is hoped, feel like continuing.

Sara coaxes the nipple into his small mouth, and, after some hesitation, a bit of formula trickles in. She sees he is holding his breath again. "C'mon, Steven, breathe. You can do more than one thing at once. C'mon." She tilts the bottle up to stop any more from entering the baby's mouth. After a moment, Steven swallows the formula and takes a breath. Sara looks at his monitor: Sats are holding. Steven is hesitating, seeming to absorb this new experience, this drinking without feeling as if he is about to die from the effort. He sucks some more and swallows, then takes a breath. It's working: He's learning what he should have known before he was born. His brain is making the connection with his senses. He is beginning to turn the corner.

A few days later, after a few more sessions with Sara Masur, Steven is beginning to feed with gusto—for the nurses and, a short time later, for Monique. At times he is pokey with the bottle, and he tires easily, sometimes before finishing, but nobody is talking food aversion anymore. His improvement is gradual but obvious. Sara's work with him is through, and another landmark in Steven's development has been achieved. First he went off the vent. Then off IVs. Soon he will be "nippling all feeds," as the nurses call it. That leaves only one more corner to turn.

"With a little luck," Jose Perez tells Monique Hachigan, "Steven will be home in just a couple more weeks."

25

THE NICU EXISTS TO TAKE CARE OF SICK INFANTS, ART STRAUSS LIKES to say, but the neonatologists exist to go to meetings.

They begin at seven in the morning and continue throughout the day, an endless parade of hospital task forces, quality control committees, peer review committees, ethics committees. If it is proposed that the unit change the way the intravenous feeding solutions are formulated, then there has to be a meeting, a study, several more meetings, more discussion. Sometimes, meetings threaten to commandeer every minute of the neonatologists' days. This week is especially bad.

For starters, there's discharge planning. Once a week, the NICU doctors, the nurse coordinators, the unit manager, the social workers, the home health nurses and a host of others gather in the NICU conference room to decide what kind of follow-up care should be given to each baby after he or she goes home.

This is not a last-minute process, cobbled together on the final day or two of a baby's stay. It begins as soon as the baby is admitted. Elias Allman's name came up for discharge planning during his first week in the unit, before anyone really knew what was wrong with him. But a plan must be in place, waiting for the day when—or if—it can be put into action. The process is almost a reverse of Morning Rounds, starting with the least sick babies and ending with the worst.

Most of the time, discharge planning is dry, uneventful, devoid of controversy. A follow-up developmental clinic will be selected for one child, an in-home program for another, a heart clinic for a third. Most of these decisions are formulaic: Children sufficiently premature or born below a certain low birth weight qualify for one program of intensive therapy and surveillance, while heartier preemies get fewer services. Brain, heart and lung diseases all trigger different programs. Sometimes discharge planning includes counseling for the parents; sometimes it goes beyond that, when abuse, neglect or drugs are suspected. A graduate from the NICU is never turned out into the world without support, some of it mandated by insurance companies or the government—a kind of protection of their half-million-dollar investment in getting the child out the door—some of it arranged by the staff not because it is being paid for, but because the child needs it. Every baby and family in the NICU is assigned a case manager, whose role is to make sure patients get every benefit and every dime they are due from insurance companies and the government, whether it's money to cover physical therapy, access to prescription drugs, or a baby-sitter so that a single mom providing round-the-clock care for a disabled preemie can get a break now and then. It makes good economic sense for the hospital to provide this service—it ensures reimbursements for the medical center, too—but there is more to it than that. Several of the case managers were neonatal nurses themselves, and they can be relentless when constructing a post-NICU safety net for those who need it most, doggedly pursuing insurers in ways no layperson could muster.

Sometimes discussions revolve less around safety nets and more around why a child *isn't* nearing discharge. In these cases, the normally placid meeting can get heated. So it is with Baby Melissa.

Melissa is the oldest baby in the unit, now coming up on her seventh month. She suffered from omphalocele, a variation of the same problem that afflicted Nikkol Hawkshaw, in which her intestines formed outside the body *in utero.* The damage was repaired, but Melissa's lungs were badly damaged in the process. She has been on a ventilator her whole life and is nowhere close to coming off—a throwback to the old days before surfactant, when many more children ended up like her. She is bloated from months on IV nourishment; her liver function is poor, her skin yellow and jaundiced. Because of the ventilator, her development is increasingly impaired. She cannot use her voice, cannot cough or chew or laugh, cannot learn to crawl or scoot or even stand.

Complicating this picture is her extreme fragility: The slightest disturbance, even changing her diaper, sends Melissa into a death dive. She literally had to be coded over a wet diaper. Strangers scare her, sending her into a spiral of asphyxiation, and so she is kept in a crib in an isolation room at one end of Room 276, normally reserved for children with contagious airborne infections. She sees only her mother, her doctors, and a few familiar nurses who have become her "primaries"—nurses who always care for a particular patient when they're on duty.

But despite all her problems, Melissa is bright and eager to learn. She loves her videos and music. Her mother, a nurse whose husband has been abroad for months with a sick parent, is unflagging in her belief that Melissa will make it. She keeps a photo album of Melissa's days in the NICU, including the horrifying birth pictures showing the enormity of the tiny baby's birth defect, which required five surgeries to correct. "I keep this book for her because someday she is going to ask me what happened," her mother says. "And I will show her." The book is entitled *Sweet Memories*.

The NICU staff is now at odds over what should happen next. She is not progressing, not getting closer to discharge, and the nurses who care for her are upset at the neonatologists. There are sixteen people in the conference room to consider this problem. The meeting was called after Melissa's mother flew into a panic when Art Strauss expressed concern that the NICU, designed for the needs of newborns, was not a proper environment for a growing baby, who needed more stimulation than the NICU could provide, room to play and develop as she approached her toddler stage. "Perhaps we should consider moving her to the Pediatric Intensive Care Unit," he had suggested. The PICU is for seriously ill older children and is something of an in-house rival of the NICU, as they both claim jurisdiction over older babies like Melissa.

"The mom is really, really concerned about this," one of the unit social workers says at the start of the meeting. "She does not want to go to Peds."

"Well, it wasn't a threat or anything," Art says defensively. "It was just a thought. She's a big child in a claustrophobic environment. Peds might be more appropriate."

Melissa's nurses weigh in then, clearly upset. They have become very attached to the girl, who, despite her many ailments, is a sweet child, able to communicate amazingly well with an arch of her eyebrows or a movement of her eyes. The nurses are not going to give her up without a fight.

"We've bonded with her," one of her primary nurses says. "And she's bonded to us. Throwing her up to Peds would be terrible for her."

Penny Jacinto sides with the nurses, uncomfortable with the idea of transferring a patient before she is well. "We've never done this before with a baby. Are we at the point . . . are we just giving up?"

"No," Art says, "my point is only that the NICU is not developmentally appropriate for a child this age. Just because we've had birthday parties here for children in the past doesn't make it appropriate."

Denise Callahan, the nurse coordinator on duty today, suggests that the real issue isn't where Melissa is treated but who is doing the treating. "What the mom really wants is a primary physician," Denise says, looking at the neonatologists one by one. "Is anyone willing to be that?"

The conference room falls silent. Denise has hit on a sensitive subject and one of the few points of contention between the NICU nurses and doctors. Nurses routinely become primaries, but not the doctors. In years past, there were primary physicians for the chronic cases, but that was when more attending physicians were available. Now the system of rotating the six attendings through the NICU's various rooms means that a different neonatologist sees the babies in each room every week. Usually, it's not an issue. But for Melissa, with her long stay and lack of progress, it has become a sore spot. The mother wants to be able to see the same doctor every time.

When none of the neonatologists responds, the primary nurse explodes: "You guys all have different plans for her. Art says, let's give her Decadron"—a steroid used to improve lung function. "Then Jose comes in and says, what's with the Decadron? And he changes it. Then the next week it's someone else. Now it's talk of transferring her upstairs!" Tears of frustration are running down the nurse's cheeks. She does not even pretend to be detached about Melissa, whom she nearly sees as a member of her family. "It's not fair. It's not fair to *her*. I'm just sick of this!"

The doctors are surprised at this outburst. The neonatologists feel they go to great lengths to preserve continuity of care as they hand off to one another, and that any discrepancies are easily worked out. Denise agrees with that, but tries a different argument: "We get complaints from parents all the time about this. Wouldn't you, as a parent, want one face, one familiar physician?"

Lupe is blunt: "No. We've been through this before. The goal is to provide a *plan* for the patient, not a person. The important thing is a care plan we all respect." A little anger creeps into her tone. She wonders if it is the nurses rather than the parents who are the sources of these complaints. "We introduce ourselves to the parents and say, you'll get to meet the six of us. How are they even getting this idea of primary care?"

"They pass the crisis, and after a week they want one doctor, like on the outside," the social worker says. "Nobody has to give them the idea. It's only natural."

"But this is different," Art says. "Outside she's not getting critical care. With our schedule, as a general rule, it's not practical. We provide the best care by rotating. Assigning individual patients would be unworkable—what do we do when we're on administrative weeks, or on vacation? It's impossible!"

The discussion grows increasingly heated, with both sides digging in, not over turf or profits or ego but over differing visions of how best to help a child get well. Parents never see these exchanges, but perhaps they should; the passion and fervor everyone in the room feels for Melissa, for all the patients in the NICU, is palpable.

At this impasse Lupe intervenes to diffuse the argument: "Let's cut to the chase. How many in this room think that the best thing for Melissa, for getting her out of this hospital, is getting her the same physician every day? Can I see a show of hands?"

She has cleverly altered the terms of the debate, for the ultimate goal, after all, is to make the girl well—to send her home. No hands go up. Lupe looks satisfied. "How many think the best thing for Melissa is having the same plan, a good plan, and getting her home?"

There are nods and murmurs and raised hands, some of them reluctant but raised nevertheless. Chastened, the primary nurse says, "Well, yes, that's what we want."

And with that the group comes together, as it always does. Nurses and doctors agree to disagree on the subject of primary physicians and to pursue a plan for the little girl they can all agree upon and carry out consistently, no matter who is in the room with Melissa.

The decision: Getting Melissa out of the NICU is now more essential than getting her off the ventilator. But the goal will be for her to go home, not to the pediatric ward. They will propose to her mother that she be given a tracheotomy—a surgical hole in her throat—through which her ventilator can pump her oxygen supply, freeing her mouth from the prison of the breathing tube. Once she has the "trake," Melissa can be switched to a less powerful portable home ventilator. She can start to eat baby food. She can start to act more like a kid.

If it works, she can go home.

"We just have to explain, this is not for the rest of her life," Lupe reminds everyone. Most parents are horrified at first by the notion of a trake. "Once she gets home, she could do better. Her lungs could regenerate . . ."

Lupe trails off. No one has to finish the thought; they all know the alternative. Melissa could improve and come off the vent after six months or a year at home, or she could gradually get worse and succumb to lung disease. Or her heart could give out from the strain of being on a vent so long. But even if that happens, she will at least know what it is like to be home. It's all they can offer: a chance at a life.

"It's time," her primary nurse agrees. "She has to get on with her life. One way or another."

The next meeting this day is a brief one: The Four-Headed Dragon goes to lunch in the doctors' dining room. Over pasta, salads and fish with some sort of white sauce on it that no one can quite identify, the doctors discuss one of the worst crises they have faced since taking over the NICU: competition.

Although the unit is full of patients now, there are troubling signs on the horizon. There has been a huge decline in transports to the unit from other hospitals, a significant drain of patients. The smaller outlying hospitals in the Los Angeles–Orange County area that rings Memorial have been sending many of their sick babies elsewhere, due to HMO contracts, underbidding and other reasons that have little to do with the quality of medical care. The four doctors would like to turn that around.

The calculation here is simple: Fewer patients sent to the NICU mean less money for the group. The doctors are not employees of the hospital and receive no payments as members of the medical staff, which is the typical relationship between hospital and physician, one reason why being on staff is a "privilege." The NICU doctors earn their living from profits gleaned from billing patients and their insurers for physician services, a separate set of charges from those billed by the hospital. Every time a patient is transported to a rival NICU, the Four-Headed Dragon loses thousands of dollars—or tens of thousands, depending on the patient.

There are many competitors targeting patients who normally would go to the NICU at Miller Children's Hospital. One rival NICU has been dispatching doctors and nurses throughout the region to give free lectures, in-service training and to attend problem deliveries at small hospitals—and, of course, to accept preemies or other ill newborns who might otherwise have been shipped to Miller Children's. Last year, Jose, Art, Lupe and Penny cut back on their own, similar marketing and outreach efforts—in part because the doctors' brutal schedule leaves little time for it, in part because the hospital, facing its own budget shortfalls, would no longer pay nurses and RTs overtime to join in such excursions. But there is also a certain amount of complacency when you're the best in town. The rival hospital, sensing an opening, has been pushing hard to fill its beds at Miller's expense.

This baby drain has been worsened by the odd bedfellows of corporate medicine. The nonprofit foundation that owns both Long Beach Memorial and Miller Children's owns five other smaller hospitals in the region as well, several of them with their own, albeit smaller and less intensive, NICUs. It would make sense for there to be a friendly relationship between these smaller neonatal units and the big NICU at Miller, but common sense does not always apply in the feverish world of medical acquisitions. When Memorial bought these smaller hospitals, some of their NICUs were being run by physician groups or large corporations in competition with the neonatologists at Miller. Their own hospital is, in effect, aiding the unit's rivals.

The doctors have been casting about for ways to counter this problem, from mass mailings extolling their NICU's virtues, to pushing the hospital to revive plans to remodel the unit, to offering to attend high-risk deliveries at community hospitals, providing a backstop where there normally is no neonatologist on duty. Medically, this last is a great idea, a potential lifesaver, but practically speaking, it's an iffy proposition. Smaller hospitals are under terrible financial strain, with more going under or being bought out every year. Delivering babies is one of their most profitable activities, making them reluctant to call in a crew of outsiders who not only will take away the baby and all its billable expenses once it arrives but who might decide to scoop up the mother before she even delivers. There's a reason why there are few such "maternal transports," despite universal agreement that they are medically advisable: The pressure to keep the patient and make the money is just too great. The smaller hospitals will give up high-risk deliveries only in the most extreme cases and even then may not err on the side of caution. They will keep the patients, deliver the babies, and hope for the best, knowing that nine times out of ten, they will be okay.

Declining transports, however, pale next to a second, more serious crisis facing the Dragon: the corporate wooing of the perinatology group that handles all the high-risk pregnancies and deliveries at Memorial. This nationally renowned group, consistently ranked among the best in the country, is a primary source of babies for the NICU, for high-risk pregnancies often produce sick or premature babies. The perinatologists have a long-standing and close relationship with the four neonatologists, but that could change quicker than the stock market should there be a buyout.

Two large medical corporations are interested in acquiring the perinatal practice; both of them, at one time or another, have expressed interest in taking over the NICU as well. One of these companies, the neonatologists believe, would probably continue the current good-neighbor policy of sending all its babies over.

The other could pose a big problem: Once in place in the women's hospital, this company—Pediatrix, the same outfit that had tried to buy the doctors out in the past—could easily decide to bring its own neonatologists to the hospital. It would then be a simple matter to refer all the babies to itself, leaving the Four-Headed Dragon out in the cold.

This dire possibility clearly weighs on the doctors. They could always find work elsewhere, their careers would continue and even flourish—that's not the issue. The threat isn't just about money. They've invested so much of themselves in this NICU for so long that leaving would be the medical equivalent of losing the family farm. For all the long hours and annoyances, each of them knows they'll never have it this good again if they have to leave.

If they did have to look elsewhere for work, the foursome would almost certainly have to break up. They might never again enjoy the autonomy they have now, the ability to practice neonatology the way they see fit, rather than according to the protocols and fiscal policies of some parent corporation. The allure of their independence cannot be underestimated in an era when medical doctors are retiring and quitting in droves and many who remain see their traditional status as captains of the ship with absolute medical authority eclipsed by the higher powers of HMOs, medical accountants, risk managers and lawyers. Much of the charting and reporting is done not to satisfy any medical purpose but to satisfy the lawyers, to safeguard against lawsuits. Going corporate would, in the minds of the neonatologists, make such concerns paramount.

There's not a lot to do at this point, the doctors know. All they can do is wait to see how everything shakes out, a helpless position they are not accustomed to.

"I try not to think about it too much," Jose Perez says later as he roots through a picked-over box of chocolates in the coordinator's office. "We can't do anything about it anyway. We'll just keep our fingers crossed. And if we have to go to war, well, we've been there, done that, too. I think we'll be okay. The Four-Headed Dragon has always managed to survive somehow."

There are several family conferences every week. These impromptu meetings are called so that the neonatologists, the nurses, a social worker, and any specialists involved in a case can meet with parents to resolve questions or problems or chart a course for the future.

Sometimes the conference is requested by the parents, as in an upcoming meeting with the Hawkshaws, who continue to be frustrated at Nikkol's lack of progress. Or they can be initiated by the staff, out of concern for the child—or the parent. The conference with the mother of Baby Girl Jones is a particularly unpleasant example of the latter.

Little Jessica Jones is perhaps the most depressing case in the NICU today. She is beautiful, full-term, chubby and perfect. She was destined to be healthy and strong, should never have seen the inside of the NICU—but for the massive hit of cocaine her mother took during labor, which had the predictable effect of destroying most of her brain.

Mom had heard that a good hit of coke could speed along delivery and spare her some pain. It speeded things along, all right: The drug caused a severe reduction in blood flow to the placenta, followed by a full-out placental abruption—a tearing away of the lifegiving placenta from the uterine wall that caused extensive bleeding. This had little lasting effect on the mother but did devastating and irreversible damage to the baby. A crash C-section was performed at the hospital in a desperate attempt to save the baby. Now only autonomic functions controlled by the most primitive part of the brain are left, which is why Baby Girl Jones could be revived at birth. Only later did the neonatologists realize what they had revived: Jessica had been asphyxiated inside her mother, as efficiently as if Mom had smothered the baby with a pillow in her crib. The only difference is that under the law, smothering a baby with a pillow is murder; destroying the child with drugs *in utero* is simply a bad choice.

The damage to Jessica's brain is called global ischemia. It affects both the higher cortical areas, the seat of intelligence, personality and memory, and the brain stem, where basic bodily functions are controlled. Global ischemia is different from a brain bleed and in many ways worse—it is a starving of the tissues of the brain that leaves whole swaths dead and atrophied.

The consequences of this are almost too numerous to describe: Jessica had severe seizures during her first day of life. None of her bodily systems worked properly, not even her ability to regulate her body temperature, because her brain could not deliver the proper commands to her muscles, organs or blood vessels. A tube was surgically inserted into

221

her belly to allow feeding—she cannot as yet suck or swallow and may never be able to do so. She is breathing and peeing and processing the nourishment pumped into her belly, which means her body can be sustained for quite some time, three or four years perhaps. But her life will have profound limits: She will never be able to speak or to understand the images and sounds that her senses perceive. She will not walk or move in any purposeful way, or know her name, or feel joy or love or sadness. She will have only pain and instinctual reactions. She will not live so much as exist, devoid of personality or will.

When Lupe brought the resident and fellow by during rounds just before the family conference, they reviewed the extensive treatment plan to keep the child's heart, lungs and digestive system going. Then the neonatologist said, "And if you're wondering why are we doing all this, when this baby already has lost the most important part of herself, the answer is, you do it because this baby's going to live. And we need to make her as comfortable as possible. And you don't want her to live forever in the hospital. So you do what you have to do." Then Lupe paused and could not conceal the bitterness in her voice. "And I am just sick of these cases, that this is still going on."

"Can't we report it to the police?" the resident asked.

"We do. We're required to by law. But no one does anything about it. Prosecutors won't touch it. They say it's not abuse until *after* the child is born."

The family conference has been called to explain the baby's dire condition to the mother. The hope is that, once explained, Mrs. Jones will sign a DNR so that nothing will be done to resuscitate Jessica should she take a turn for the worse and code. Although it galls the nurses caring for Jessica, the mother still calls the shots on this score. Were the NICU to withhold treatment without the mother's permission, she could sue—and conceivably profit handsomely from the human disaster she herself had caused.

In the conference room, Penny and a consulting neurologist patiently explain the injury to Jessica's brain, her poor prognosis, the near certainty that a vegetative existence is all the child will ever experience. At best, assuming no setbacks, Jessica will probably live only a handful of years—with around-the-clock care. The social worker is almost coddling Mrs. Jones, telling her she needs to look out for herself, get counseling, move on. And then they ask her what she wants done if Jessica codes. Does Mrs. Jones want CPR, code drugs, the works next time? Or will she authorize a DNR?

"No, I want everything done. I want you to do everything to save my baby, whatever it takes," the teary-eyed Mrs. Jones says. "I want to have the chance to apologize to her, to tell her how sorry I am."

Mrs. Jones's sister, herself a nurse who has come in from out of town and has remained silent until now, suddenly speaks. "No," she says, looking Mrs. Jones in the eye, her words slow but angry, "you've got to let her go and get yourself into a drug program. If you're really sorry, like you say you are, that's what you'll do."

Mrs. Jones is still shaking her head stubbornly. The social worker adds, "I know this is tough for you. This is a new experience. You need some time . . ."

The sister interrupts. She is livid now, looking directly at Mrs. Jones, who is hanging her head, unwilling to meet her sister's eyes. "Didn't you tell them?" She turns to the others again. "This isn't new. Twenty months ago, the same thing happened. She knows. She wanted everything done then, too, but the little boy died after twenty weeks. It was awful."

The people in the conference room are left gape-mouthed at this revelation, trying to absorb the fact that this is the second baby whose brain was destroyed by this woman's drug use. Somehow, this was omitted from the medical history—perhaps because it took place in another state, and such things aren't tracked in any systematic way. The doctors rely on the parents to provide an accurate history; the father is out of the picture in this case, and the mother, unsurprisingly, said nothing of her last baby as she sought to portray herself as an infrequent drug user who had simply made a mistake. Nor did she mention the three other cocaine-addicted babies she had previously delivered, babies who survived but who have lifelong problems. The sister tells the gathering, though, explaining how she is raising one of the children herself—he is standing next to her, a fidgeting three-year-old everyone assumed was her own child. "I just can't go through this again," the sister says. "I just can't. It's got to stop." Yet Mrs. Jones, through her tears, still insists she wants everything done for Jessica, no matter what.

The enormity of the evil she has done is now clear: Knowing that her drug use had harmed her other children, and that it had profoundly damaged and killed the last, she has still destroyed yet another life. The mother is looking down at her hands, shaking her head—not denying it, but just not wanting to hear or acknowledge the ugly truth. She has decided, through the twisted logic of a drug abuser, that she will make amends by defending her baby's meager life, however belatedly and cruelly. She does not look or sound like a drug addict even now. She is clean, she has a job, she is educated. But for the first time, the people around the table are looking at her as if she were a monster.

The conference seems to have reached an impasse on this awful, uncomfortable note. But Debbie Evans, the child's nurse, who was already stewing quietly beneath her professional demeanor, who has held this baby in her arms and felt her lifelessness, can barely contain herself now. She is an imposing woman, not known for suffering in silence, gentle and patient most times but forceful, even blunt, when circumstances call for it. And when she hears the social worker begin to repeat her assertion that Mrs. Jones's priority should be looking out for herself and getting counseling, Debbie finally can restrain herself no longer.

"I think I know what's going on here. You feel guilty for what you chose to do nine months ago," she says with quiet force. "The thing is, your baby will not know your apology. She will never know your touch or your voice. She is going to live in foster care because of what you did to her. If you really love your baby, you will not let her suffer anymore. You will stop this."

Mrs. Jones was wailing before Debbie has finished, but the nurse could not stop herself once she had begun. The tough talk has the desired effect: Mrs. Jones sobs, "I know. I know I did this. I know."

Debbie looks around at the others at the conference. One person flashes her a thumbs-up under the table. The sister is nodding in agreement. And the social worker says, "We will help you get into a drug program." Mrs. Jones nods. The meeting ends on a positive note of sorts, if such a thing is possible in this awful case.

In the end, though, Mrs. Jones sticks by her guns. There will be no DNR. Clinically, the baby is not brain-dead, and therefore there are no grounds for the NICU to go to court and ask for an order superseding the mother's wishes. Jessica's life will be maintained no matter what until she can be sent home to a pointless existence, a life filled with pain and a mother's apologies she'll never comprehend.

The one meeting the neonatologists want to pull off but have been unable to do is a family conference about Nikkol Hawkshaw. "We need to do something for them—and for this baby," her primary nurse, Nancy Burkey, told Penny Jacinto one afternoon. "She isn't going anywhere, and they're frustrated. And I don't blame them."

Penny agreed to do what she could, but getting the necessary players together proved challenging. Stuart Hawkshaw is a driver for United Parcel Service—he met his wife, Kristine, making a delivery to the doctor's office where she works—and December is his busiest month. He cannot take time off from work to meet at the hospital. He asked for a nighttime meeting, which the neonatologists, social workers and nurses were happy to oblige. But the GI doctors, the gastrointestinal specialists who are trying to jump-start Nikkol's failing intestines and liver, were no-shows. They are too busy for after-hours meetings.

The Hawkshaws were furious. They complained to Nancy that, not only could they not meet with the GI docs, their calls were never returned, either. Nancy passed this on to Art, who was inclined to give his colleagues the benefit of the doubt—until he had to call them several times before getting a response. The neonatologists don't like being caught in the middle, and Art made it clear that both he and the Hawkshaws expected action. "We've just been swamped," he was told. "But we'll get something set up right away."

Finally, another meeting was called. One of the GI physicians would come to do an endoscopy of Nikkol—placing a fiber-optic cable inside her stomach, literally to have a look around. Then he would attempt to place a jejunal feeding tube—a way of bypassing the stomach, another part of Nikkol's anatomy that was badly damaged, and putting food directly into her small intestine. The hope was that this would get her digestive system moving, since the feeding tube to her stomach was doing nothing but breeding bacteria. An infectious disease specialist would be on hand to figure out what role if any the infection was playing in Nikkol's digestive problems. Most important, it would be done when Stuart was off, so he could be there for the procedure. It would not be a full-blown family conference, but it would be something. And the Hawkshaws needed to see at least some sign of progress.

There had been one other bit of progress: Nikkol was in Room 276 now, finally off the ventilator, although no one knew how long that would last. Her lungs were weak and damaged, but the primary problem remained her inability to feed. That problem needed to be solved very soon.

Stuart appears for the endoscopy red-eyed and exhausted, but relieved that something is being done. His daughter has been in the Long Beach NICU for eight weeks, transferred from a hospital in Torrance where she was born and spent her first three months. She was transferred because the surgeon who performed the five original gastroschisis surgeries wanted Visut Kanchanapoom's assistance for additional surgery. Nikkol had developed strictures in her intestines—scar tissue that blocked off the flow and made digestion impossible. She ending up losing 80 percent of her small intestine during this final operation, leaving precious little to survive on.

In the meantime, five months of intravenous feedings have taken their toll on Nikkol's liver, leaving her almost orange with jaundice, as if she has been painted. Without a functioning digestive process in which her liver can flush itself of toxins, the damage to that crucial organ continues and may soon become irreversible.

"It'll be a miracle if this girl survives," Stuart suddenly blurts, as he stares at the sleeping form of his daughter. He instantly feels guilty for saying such a thing. "I'm just so stressed, so tired. So worried about Kris."

His eyes are locked on his daughter, and the words just tumble out of him: "They tell you this is going to be a roller coaster, but nothing prepares you for this. Every week we get our hopes up again. 'We're starting her feeds again,' they tell us. And every time, our hopes are dashed. It's her bowels, it's her liver, it's her lungs, it's always something holding her back. I mean, Kris puts her head on the pillow some nights and cries all night. I go to work, and people ask, 'How's Nikkol? Oh, she's *still* in the hospital?' Over and over. And you just grit your teeth. And they ask, 'How can you stand it?' Like I have a choice."

The Hawkshaws have reached a point in the NICU experience few parents know anymore, a harkening back to the old days, when it was not so unusual for six months or a year to pass before a child with chronic illnesses like Nikkol's could make it home. Stuart and Kristine have stopped going out as a couple. Stuart has a five-year-old daughter and an eight-year-old son from a previous marriage, and they adore Kris, but they have stopped doing things together. If they want to go to a movie or play a board game—things their stepmom always did with them before—she says no, she has to make some calls about Nikkol or go over medical bills for Nikkol or read up on some new treatment possibility for Nikkol. Stuart knows this is how his wife deals with her helplessness, by trying to do something, anything. But the kids don't understand. They want Nikkol to come home, but they don't miss her because they have never had her. The person they miss is Kris. As does Stuart.

Nancy Burkey always makes it a point to talk to Stuart, to ask him how things are going at home. She is a quiet woman for the most part, but when she does express her opinion, she is direct, cutting to the heart of the matter—which in this case is preserving a young family from destruction. Nancy knows that the stress of having a chronically ill infant is hell on marriages; half the couples who have such children end up breaking up, no matter how things turn out for the baby. So she gently prods Stuart into talking openly about his feelings, which are much more pessimistic than his wife's. He has begun to wonder if they have gone too far with Nikkol.

"She is in such pain all the time, she looks so miserable, she's so far away from healthy, I just don't know anymore," he confesses. "I wonder if I'll ever get to see her in a crib at home, if I'll ever push her in a swing at the playground. But I can't say that to Kris. I'm afraid to say it to myself."

The GI doctor arrives, providing a welcome return to more tangible things: the ins and outs of the procedure he's performing, how the new feeding tube will work, what they hope to accomplish. Then Stuart watches as the physician places a long, flexible black tube down Nikkol's throat. The end of the tube inside Nikkol has a light and a magnifying lens; its intense brightness can be seen shining pinkly through Nikkol's belly. The other end of the tube has an eyepiece and a focusing knob, which the doctor moves around as if he were a fisherman reeling in a catch, an odd marriage of high tech gadgetry and the low-tech push and pull of a plumber's snake. He jerks the tube to one side and gets a clear view of Nikkol's stomach. It looks bad, he says, like raw hamburger. It should look like the pink interior of a healthy mouth. It is aswarm with bacteria. Not good.

He pushes the tube in further, then moves the eyepiece around until the small intestines come into focus. Much better, he says. They're small but healthy and pink. No signs of infection. Now he works the jejunal tube into place, which involves a lot more pushing and pulling. Nancy asks Stuart if he's okay—it's an ugly procedure to watch, and Nikkol has had to be heavily sedated to keep from coding from the pain. But Stuart, face set with grim resolve, says, "I watched all the reduction surgeries. She's my daughter. I'm okay."

After about fifteen minutes, the tube is placed. The doctor then inflates a small balloon at its tip, which will anchor it beyond the stomach. "In a day, we can start feeds," he says. "And we'll keep our fingers crossed."

When the doctor from the hospital's infectious disease department steps in, Stuart asks him if he can do something to knock out all those bacteria infecting Nikkol's stomach. The answer surprises him: The doctor says he wants to keep Nikkol off antibiotics as much as possible.

"At this point we wouldn't be killing the bacteria, we'd just be choosing which organisms you'll have in there. The problem is that the gut isn't working. If it was, those bacteria wouldn't be there."

"But the reason it's not working is the infection," Stuart objects.

The doctor nods. It is a classic catch-22: Nikkol's stomach is infected because it isn't working. And it won't work as long as it's infected.

The solution, the doctor says, may lie in the jejunal tube. If it works and food starts flowing through the intestines, the stomach may start functioning as well, and then the bacteria will begin to die. She can come off IV nutrition, and her liver will get a chance to heal. "At least, that's our hope."

Stuart looks at him. "Your hope?"

"What I'm saying is, no promises."

After he leaves, Stuart mutters, "No promises. What's new?"

The jejunal tube seems to work for a few days, but then it, too, begins to back up. Nikkol is put back on NPO status. Then she begins to shows signs of infection. Soon she is back on the ventilator and back in Room 288. Back to where she started.

There is another meeting this week, the strangest one of all. It takes place not in the conference room or cafeteria but deep in the bowels of the hospital, down near the morgue, in the pathology department.

Lupe, Pure and Dr. Leonel Guajardo, the latest addition to the ranks of the neonatal attendings, have been invited to make this unusual pilgrimage. After a long walk through echoing hallways, they step beyond an electronically locked door to a complex of rooms that appears to be a cross between a mad scientist's laboratory and an accountant's office. It is crammed with files, ledgers and books, as well as shelf after shelf of specimen jars filled with tissue samples and human organs swimming darkly in solutions of preservative.

They are here to resolve the mystery of Baby Girl Angela McGee.

Angela was born a few weeks earlier. The head of the pediatric heart program at the hospital had come by the NICU to let the attendings know a baby was about to be delivered three weeks premature with an abnormally enlarged heart, one that appeared so huge on fetal ultrasound that treatment, perhaps surgery, would have to be very swift. Plans were laid for the baby to be stabilized and brought to the NICU for an immediate echocardiogram by the hospital's top heart ultrasound specialist, Mary Jo Barnes, a frequent and much-valued visitor to the unit, renowned for her ability to interpret the eerie sonic images her machine produces. Normally the heart echo is done later, but for this baby, Mary Jo would come by immediately.

A few hours later, the call came over the Stentofon, summoning a neonatal team to the labor and delivery room where Angela was to be born. Pure arrived just in time to be handed a squalling, blond-haired, pink-skinned beauty who looked perfectly healthy, if a little small. She was vigorous, kicking, with good color and a lusty cry, with her Apgar score initially at eight, then rising to nine in five minutes—as good as most healthy newborns'. Pure put her stethoscope to the baby's chest, ready to hear that huge heart straining inside, but it sounded normal: no murmur, no rattle. Everything sounded fine, except for some odd breath sounds. Maybe there was a problem with the lungs—they'd do an X ray right away back at the unit, a matter of routine—but the heart seemed normal. This was the NICU's favorite sort of delivery—a baby not nearly as sick as believed.

Back at the unit, the echocardiogram confirmed Pure's impression of Angela's heart: Mary Jo could find little or nothing wrong with it. The obstetrician who delivered Angela came in, still in full surgical regalia, having just finished dealing with the mother's afterbirth and initial recovery. "The mom's on pins and needles," the OB said. "What can I tell her?"

"Tell her it looks like the heart's pretty much normal," the cardiologist, who had been peering over Mary Jo's shoulder, said. "Tell her that she can relax, that these guys here in the NICU will be taking over now."

The OB dashed back to her patient with the happy news. But it was not to last. When Pure and Leonel went downstairs to check the chest X rays, they immediately saw why the normal heart had appeared so large on the fetal ultrasound: It looked huge compared to the baby's lungs. Angela's lungs were stunted, barely developed. Hypoplastic lung, the condition is called, a rare and grave condition because the lungs can be so small that they cannot support life.

For the next several hours, Pure, Leonel and Clyde Mori, one of the unit's most experienced respiratory therapists, worked to save Angela. But no matter what they did, her pink, healthy skin gradually turned pale, then gray, as her insufficient lungs failed to give her body enough oxygen.

Still, they were not prepared to give up. This was not something they saw very often, and almost never in a child who had emerged from the womb appearing so healthy. And so they used enormous pressures on the ventilator, hoping that the lungs might expand like underinflated balloons. When that failed, they switched her off and on every kind of ventilator they had—jet, conventional, oscillator—in the hope of finding the right match. They used every drug they had that can improve respiratory function. When those tactics failed, Leonel called different experts in neonatal pulmonology. Could the same nitric oxide treatment that had benefited Baby Girl Berger be of help here? Or could Angela benefit from extra corporeal membrane oxygenation—a controversial and difficult use of a modified heart-lung machine that would bypass the baby's lungs and put oxygen into the blood without her having to breathe?

Leonel was loath to give up, but finally he hung up the phone, dispirited. Nothing worked, and nothing would work. Even under fantastic ventilator pressures and rates, with 100 percent oxygen, Angela's sats kept falling little by little. Her chest barely moved, Clyde observed, like a block of wood—there was next to nothing in there for the ventilator to fill and empty. He put his hand on her chest and said, "I can't feel a thing. Her chest should be bouncing like crazy now, but it isn't budging an inch."

"If there're no lungs there, then there're no lungs there. No treatment we use is going to change that," Leonel reluctantly said. They had run out of options. It was time to break the news to Angela's parents— dashing hopes that had been so cruelly raised when the baby's heart had turned out to be all right.

"These are the times when this is the worst job in the world," Kathy Hauck, Angela's nurse, said, her eyes red. "You always feel like you want to do more. Usually we can. Today we can't."

When she received the news, Angela's mother rocked and kissed her new baby and begged Leonel to give explanations he did not possess.

"We don't know why this happens," he replied honestly. "Something in the baby didn't develop. We just don't know."

"What if we just waited three weeks and gave her lungs a chance to grow?" the father asked Lupe later, desperation on his face as his three-year-old son screamed and clung to his leg. He had rushed to the hospital, unable to find a last-minute baby-sitter, unaware of the dire turn of events until the moment he walked into the room.

The night coordinator, Martha Rivera, offered to watch the little boy out in the hall, and Lupe turned to Mr. McGee, reviewing all the things that had been done and considered for his daughter. "And yes, there may be ways to prolong her life," she said, "but I'm very sorry, no, her lungs are not going to grow. Ever. In the end, nothing we do is going to change that." And then everyone in the unit had to see that look steal across the young couple's faces, the look no parent should ever have to wear. They asked for a priest so their daughter could be baptized. And then they signed the papers authorizing the withdrawal of life support for their new baby.

A few hours later, in the privacy of one of the small family rooms, Angela was removed from the ventilator and carried to her parents and brother, who held her and petted her and watched her die. Ironically, the heart everyone had believed to be so damaged proved so strong and hearty that it kept Angela alive for twenty more minutes before finally giving out.

Now, a little more than two weeks later, the doctors have trooped down to the basement to meet with the pathologist in his odd domain. He takes them in back and pulls out a gray specimen of some sort on a small tray. It looks like a fossil, ancient, the color of parchment. He picks it up and holds it carefully, almost reverentially, in his gloved hands.

He is holding Angela McGee's heart and lungs.

"You see here," the pathologist is saying, "the entire trachea and esophagus were constricted. There was an anomalous blood vessel that wound around it and inhibited growth."

The parents had authorized a chest-only autopsy of their day-old girl—they wanted to know more about what had happened to her, and so did her doctors. The neonatologists believed they had done everything they could, and yet . . . good doctors always question themselves, always acknowledge their fears, always want to know just what they were up against. So they peer at this poor girl's organs, feeling ill at ease. They are trained as scientists, and all of them have seen cadavers and organs before, yet there is something profoundly disquieting about being here, about handling this particular heart and lungs from a baby they had tried so desperately to save. The mood is somber; they feel like strangers at a wake.

They see clearly what the pathologist is pointing out. Something happened very early in Angela's embryonic development, some part of that complex unfolding from egg to human that went awry: An out-of-place blood vessel had wrapped itself like a boa constrictor around the baby's windpipe and lungs, strangling them, keeping them from growing properly. That was why the ventilator had done no good: Not only were the lungs too small, but the windpipe through which the air had to pass was no wider than the metal wire in a paper clip. The doctors had been right, the pathologist assures them: No treatment or surgery or procedure could have altered the fundamental flaw in Angela's respiratory system. Her condition was irreversible and incompatible with life. It is also extremely rare and not likely to recur should the parents have another child.

Pure nods. "So there really was nothing we could do."

"At least the parents will know now," the pathologist adds as the doctors file out of the hushed lab. "They'll know they did the right thing."

The others murmur their assent, but no one who saw the look on the McGees' faces really believes this knowledge will make them feel the least bit better.

When they return upstairs, the Stentofon announces a routine birth in Labor and Delivery. There's just a little meconium in the amniotic fluid, a little suctioning to be done—a piece of cake for the NICU, a welcome distraction, a reminder that life continues relentlessly, sometimes in sadness, sometimes in joy. Now it's joy's turn.

26

A DAY AFTER HIS ROTO-ROOTER, ELIAS ALLMAN IS LOOKING GOOD
enough to be removed from Room 288 and rolled next door to the
step-down room.

Room 276 is a larger, quieter room with more windows and natural
light. A baby is sitting in a swing, rocking gently, trailing IVs and an
oxygen line. The kids in here are still in need of intensive care, but they
are not on the most critical list, which means the room has a calmer feel
to it; it seems almost relaxed compared to the hypervigilant environment of Room 288. Elias rolls to a stop two incubators over from Jordan Leos and just across the width of the room from Steven Hachigan.

In truth, the move was less because Elias had shown dramatic improvement—he had not—and more because there were sicker kids
who needed the most intensive care the NICU could provide. "He was
the least sick one in the room," Julie France later explains. "So I had to
move him. Kind of like when you ask for a volunteer, and everyone else
takes a step back." Nevertheless, Amalia and Robert take this "graduation" as a good omen, even after Elias's nurse carefully explains that
there are still many concerns. Chief among these is the fact that, even
after the Roto-Rooter and the easing of Elias's stomach bloat, he has yet
to have a bowel movement.

Lupe is particularly concerned by this. Her initial optimism that
Elias's problem had been solved has faded. On rounds, she asks Valerie
Josephson what Elias's symptoms might add up to, assuming the block-

age of meconium was not the underlying problem but merely a symptom of something else. She reviews Elias's main problems: his persistent air sac collapse, the condition called atelectasis; his inability to wean from the ventilator; and his unusual difficulty passing the meconium Visut flushed out. "What can that indicate?" Lupe asks her resident.

Valerie thinks a moment, then answers, "It could be CF."

"Very good. Cystic fibrosis," Lupe confirms, slipping into the role of teacher. "It can present in this way. So what do we do to test this hypothesis?"

"We need a family history," Valerie decides after a moment. "And we should order a DNA swab."

"Let's do it. And we should consider another obstructive series if he doesn't poop soon." Lupe shakes her head. "Mom is not going to be a happy camper when you start asking her about CF. Make sure she understands this test is to rule it out, not because we feel certain he has it. Poor kid."

There are aspects of medicine that are rote, a certain drug for a certain condition, a certain response to a particular finding. There are aspects that are sheer engineering—closing a PDA or excising a damaged bowel. But diagnosis is often an art, a form of enlightened theorizing— a guess, based upon symptoms, textbook parameters, a physician's experience, a gut feeling. The problem is, many diseases share the same symptoms. Elias might have a meconium plug blocking his intestines, the simplest answer and the easiest to fix. But he might also have cystic fibrosis, a genetic glandular disorder that impairs the lungs and other organs. He might have a defect that the obstructive series of X rays failed to detect. He might have another rare disease in which ganglia are missing from the lower intestines, leaving them dysfunctional and prone to blockage. The trick is finding the right test to confirm the diagnosis, then finding the right treatment for it. This is often more a process of elimination than confirmation—the same "rule-out" approach taken when infections are suspected in the NICU. Elias's problem is still a mystery, the list of suspects still too long. Tests can pare them down, however, and eventually lead to the culprit—preferably before he gets any sicker.

When the subject of cystic fibrosis is raised with Amalia that afternoon during her first visit of the day, she is shocked, just as Lupe expected. She says she knows of no one in her family with the disease, but she promises to check with her parents. Then she races to the hospital medical library for information about CF. She has heard of it, of course, but doesn't really know what it's about, other than it is one of those dreaded childhood diseases that people periodically go door to door for, collecting money in cans. She learns that it is a genetic glandular disease that primarily afflicts Caucasians, which would rule out her Filipino-Chinese heritage (though not Robert's Scotch-Irish ancestry). More important, she learns that this defect in the way the body produces mucus (particularly in the lungs) is treatable and that people with CF can lead long, happy lives. She is further relieved when she returns to the unit and the nurse reiterates that the DNA test is to *rule out* cystic fibrosis; that, absent a known history of it in the family, they don't really expect to find it. In the NICU, sometimes you have to hear things a few times before they sink in.

Amalia signs off on the test, then debates whether she should shelter Robert from this latest turn of events or tell him about it. In the end she decides to tell him. Not so much because she feels he needs to know—she'd just as soon shield him until they know more—but because she wants to question him about whether CF runs in his side of the family. He tells her no, as far as he knows. "I need to ask Mom to be sure," he says, "but we have to think about how to do it without freaking her out." Robert's mother has taken Elias's premature birth and illness every bit as hard as Amalia and Robert. All the two women have to do is sit down together, and they burst into tears. "We're waterworks, what can I say?" Amalia says apologetically whenever Robert sees them weeping in tandem.

Later, the resident takes a DNA sample from Elias by using a toothbrushlike tool to scrape cells from the inside of his cheek. The nurse tells Amalia that this procedure is quick but not entirely painless; it takes some vigorous rubbing of the delicate mucous membranes in Elias's mouth to get enough cellular material for the test. This time, Amalia decides she doesn't want to watch—the Roto-Rooter almost killed her. As it turns out, the swab was rough on Elias as well: Like so many things in the NICU, the tests and procedures vital to helping the babies also have the unintended effect of putting them through hell.

"He really got mad at us," the night-shift nurse, Karin Nakamura, reports when Amalia returns. "He wouldn't calm down afterward, and his sats really dropped. We had to give him Ativan." Ativan is a brand name for the tranquilizer lorazepam, the drug of choice in the NICU for an agitated baby, mild but effective.

Amalia rushes to Elias's incubator but sees he's asleep. She calls softly to him, using her pet name for the baby, "Boo-boo," but he doesn't react. She turns to the nurse. "When will we know the results of the test?"

Karin shakes her head. "It usually takes three to four weeks."

Amalia groans. "I wish we could know sooner than that."

Karin doesn't say anything. She's a relatively new nurse, still learning after five months on the job, but she knows enough to know that Elias isn't going to be able to wait three weeks before something has to be done about his stomach. As it turns out, Elias can't wait even three days. The nurses try to feed him, but he can't seem to digest the milk. A few hours after the feeding, his stomach is suctioned, a routine test of digestive function. In a healthy baby, only gastric juices will come up. But Elias has residual milk; in fact, almost as much comes back as he was given. It was just sitting there, curdling. He is made NPO again. Within twenty-four hours, his bowel loops are back and his stomach has again bloated. The Roto-Rooter did not do the trick.

Elias is nearly three weeks old. If he were in the womb, he would still be nine weeks from birth. Most twenty-eight-weekers are feeding by now and have left the ventilator behind. Elias can do neither. He is painfully thin, hardly over four pounds, a bare eight ounces over his birth weight. He has lines around his eyes, and his long preemie face has sunken, drawn cheeks. He looks like an old man—a very unhealthy old man, Amalia says morosely.

More X rays, ultrasounds and cultures are taken. Still nothing seems to be wrong; the bloat in his stomach appears to be just gas. Cystic fibrosis is looking more likely, but just in case, the surgeon is called for another consultation. Maybe a second Roto-Rooter will help.

It's a classic night on call for Lupe Padilla: Hectic, demanding, exhausting. One crisis seems to erupt before the previous one ends. Test results are coming back with contradictory findings. Kids are acting infected when the labs say they're fine, and infected kids are acting as if nothing's wrong.

"Everyone's acting up," a frustrated Lupe announces, standing in the middle of the room, sounding for all the world like a teacher who has lost control of her class. Pretending that crumping babies (NICU slang for babies whose sats and heart rates fall rapidly) are actually only misbehaving children, and then talking aloud to them as if they could be scolded into improving, is one of her late-night coping mechanisms. "The black cloud is the room."

Valerie, after three years of residency under Lupe, knows enough to jab a thumb in her mentor's direction. "Yeah, and there's the source of the cloud. It's like sprinkling fairy dust. In reverse."

While the resident leaves to put out fires in Room 276, where several babies are getting septic and may need more intensive care, Lupe is hopping from baby to baby in Room 288. Some nights on call can be boring, with little to do but sleep. Not tonight. David Rios is desatting and has yet another infection—every time they think he's about to turn the corner, something else seems to come in and crush him anew. He has only one functioning lung, and nobody knows how much more it can take. Nikkol Hawkshaw, meanwhile, though over her infection, refuses to come down on her ventilator settings far enough to extubate—although Lupe decides to take her off anyway, hoping to force the issue. "Something needs to happen for this kid," she says, "and if we wait for the settings, that day will never come."

But it is the Lee triplets who are consuming the bulk of Lupe's time. Each of them is showing signs of pulmonary edema and infection, yet the cultures have been negative on all but Eric. That is supposed to mean the other two have no infection, despite the symptoms. Lupe is busily ordering platelet transfusions, antibiotics and more labs on all three, trying to figure out what's going on with them or at least battle their symptoms, whether she knows their cause or not.

Osmond Lee, having recovered nicely from PDA surgery, is doing the best of the bunch. He is steadily weaning from the vent and may be off in a few days. Lupe wanted him to start feeds today, accomplished by squeezing the gavage tube past the breathing tube, but his belly was bloated and they put it off another day. "Stop being a pill," she tells the baby. "You've got to eat, child."

She picks a piece of paper just delivered—Osmond's complete blood count results—and groans, "Damn, damn, damn." The CBC is very poor, full of indicators of possible infection, and she orders more cultures. This is a problem, she tells the fellow on duty tonight, because Marlon has already received all but two antibiotics used in the NICU; one more infection will exhaust them all and create a risk of a drug-resistant bacterium taking root.

Eric Lee, who was once extubated and in Room 276, Lisa Lee's pride and joy and the triplet most everyone expected to do well, is now on the oscillator and looks awful. His entire body is puffed up from retained fluids. He hasn't peed in twenty-four hours, which means his body can't clear out built-up potassium, an element that becomes toxic to the heart once it reaches a certain level. Various infections seem to be affecting his kidneys, which forces a reluctant Lupe to cancel the best antifungal drug she has for battling his yeast infection, replacing it with a less effective medication. This is no small matter: the lowly yeast infection, a minor disease elsewhere in the hospital, is a blood-borne killer in the NICU, encouraged to grow like wildfire because the antibiotics consumed by the gallon here to keep sepsis at bay also kill many helpful background bacteria, including organisms that prey on yeast. Yeasts also thrive particularly well in the plastic tubing used by the yard to dispense IVs, waiting to reach a kind of invisible critical mass, then attacking a weakened baby full force. The antifungal drug's unfortunate side effect is its toxicity to the kidneys, something Eric can no longer afford. He is painfully swollen, his skin a dark ruddy color, and the large doses of diuretics being pumped into him intravenously are hardly making a dent. Lupe and Irene Muehlfeld the night coordinator, are working furiously, trying to find a good vein for a new IV to pump in more diuretics; his right arm is shot, and they have to flip him and move to his left. Ultimately, they have to stick a needle into his forehead in order to find a decent vein. He doesn't even react. The baby is on full life support now. Before, as with most of the kids, the ventilator *assisted* his breathing. Now it's doing all the work for Eric, a very bad sign.

Lisa Lee has come in—the nurse called her and told her she needed to be there, which is what parents are told when death may be imminent—and she is cooing at Eric, "Hi son, you're a good boy. I know you've had a bad day today. Can you open your eyes?" She sees a flicker of her son's eyelids. "Look, look, he opened an eye for me. Hi, son. I love you, son. You're a good boy. You're a strong boy."

Lupe steps back and sighs, then says softly, "It's shape-up or ship-out time, kiddo."

The third Lee brother, Marlon, is the mystery man of the night. He has all the signs of a severe infection. He has a temperature of 105. His respiration is impaired from edema—the beginning of the same problem affecting Eric. And worst of all, he is suffering from thrombocytopenia, a very low platelet count, at 19,000, a mere eighth of normal. This lack of blood-clotting factor puts him at risk of brain bleeds and other ailments.

Marlon's decline also screws up plans for him to receive the same heart surgery his brother Osmond benefited from. Lupe knows the cautious Dr. Ravelo will almost certainly refuse to operate on Marlon's PDA now, for fear of excessive bleeding. Marlon's PDA had been closed by drug treatment for a time but has now reopened. This happens sometimes in the sickliest micropreemies. Infection would be the normal suspect when platelets drop so low, but Marlon's cultures have all been negative. Now Lupe suspects a swollen liver might account for the platelet mystery, and she orders an ultrasound to confirm or rule it out. Later, she sees Mavis, the ultrasound technician, attending to another baby.

"Did you do my Baby Lee's abdomen?" she asks.

Mavis looks up. "Yes."

"Did you find anything?"

She hears eagerness in Lupe's voice and gives her a funny look. "No," she says slowly.

Lupe is exasperated. "Maaaavis," she calls plaintively.

The technician is perplexed. Negative findings are usually a good thing. "What, you wanted me to find something?"

"Yes, I wanted you to find something. If it was his liver, we could fix that." But Mavis just shakes her head. "Damn, we're missing something. But what? A virus? His PDA?"

Lupe next tries to talk Dr. Ravelo into operating on Marlon's PDA despite the low platelets. As she knew he would, the surgeon takes one look at Marlon's platelet count and balks: "Lupe, he'll never make it. Get me up to 100,000, and we'll talk."

She tries to bargain with him like a car salesman, asking him what it'll take to talk him into operating anyway. She senses Marlon needs to turn the corner soon or he never will. Sometimes changing one element of a preemie's system can affect the entire system for the better, and the PDA is one of the few things Lupe knows can be changed. "We'll give him platelets before, during and after," she says. "How about it?" But the surgeon just shakes his head: too risky for his tastes.

When he leaves, Lupe speculates that she can recruit one of the cardiologists to help her gang up on the surgeon, maybe talk him down to a platelet count of 50,000. Marlon's nurse laughs, but not out of amusement. "Yeah, I know," Lupe says. "With this kid, I might as well be asking for a million." She decides to cancel all of Marlon's antibiotics, since the tests all show he's not infected despite his symptoms. Maybe that will change the dynamics of his system for the better.

Lupe barely has set aside Marlon's chart when a nurse calls her over to see the first of twenty-seven-week twin boys admitted just a day earlier. Fragile and unstable all day, the two-day-old baby is finally crashing, as the neonatologists had feared he would. As she goes to work, Lupe sees the classic symptoms of an intraventricular hemorrhage happening right before her eyes—a bleeding in the brain she is helpless to stop because by the time it is apparent, the damage has already been done. It's those weak preemie blood vessels at work, so easily ruptured by stress, by the ventilator, by sheer gravity once outside the womb.

The baby is a ghastly shade of white, his skin papery. His blood pressure has shot through the roof. His heart rate has sagged. This is the classic aftermath of intraventricular hemorrhage. His chart—like the chart of every preemie like him in the unit—says he is at risk for a bleed. That just goes with the territory. He just happens to be one of the ones in which risk becomes reality. It happened without warning. He had actually been doing a bit better for the last hour, or so it seemed, responding to the drug dopamine, given to raise what had been dangerously low blood pressure. Now Lupe suspects his brain bleed might at least in part be an adverse reaction to that lifesaving drug.

All Lupe can do now is to try and minimize the damage. She cuts off the dopamine and replaces it with new drugs to boost his heart rate. An RT bags him to get his sats back up. After a bit, his color comes back and his vitals seem stable again. Maybe it was just a mild bleed, Lupe suggests, though only a head ultrasound can tell for sure. The quickness of the episode bodes well for him.

Ten minutes later, as Lupe makes a futile attempt to wolf down some dinner in the coordinator's office, twin number two follows in his brother's footsteps. He does exactly the same thing: The terrible pallor is there, the blood pressure skyrockets, the heart rate plummets. Lupe replays the same treatment, except this twin hadn't been getting blood pressure medicine. This one takes longer to revive, and even then his previously pink color does not return. He goes from white to a kind of sickly gray. His vitals don't improve as much as his brother's, either, and Lupe knows, even before the head ultrasound confirms it later that night, even before he starts the seizures and the stiff posturing indicative of brain damage, that he has had a much more severe bleed than his brother.

Identical twins, across the room from each other, on different drugs and unconnected in any way, have suffered the same catastrophic illness within minutes of each other.

"That is totally weird," the resident says.

"Believe it or not, we've seen this before," Lupe says. "Twins do that."

"Do we know what caused it?"

Lupe shakes her head. "Maybe the unstable blood pressure and dopamine for the first one, but this guy, we don't know. If we knew what caused it, we could stop it from happening."

Lupe checks the babies' histories. They came in by ambulance a day ago. The mother had shown up at a local community hospital's emergency room in active labor, her first and only visit to a doctor during her entire pregnancy. By then, her premature contractions, which might have been stopped with drugs had she come in sooner, could not be slowed. She was too far along to be rushed to Memorial as a maternal transport, the preferred course of action when a mother is about to deliver high-risk preemies. Instead, the twins were rushed to Memorial by ambulance immediately after birth, on ventilators and in extreme distress—a less-than-optimum situation, as bouncy ambulance rides are tolerated far better inside the womb than outside, especially if you happen to have arrived three months before your scheduled birth date.

Lupe can see from the medical history in the chart that the mother, who is still hospitalized across town where she gave birth, should have understood the value of prenatal care: She already has a three-year-old and a seven-month-old and so can have no reasonable excuse for her neglect. The twins' prematurity and critical condition could probably have been made less serious, if not avoided entirely, by a more responsible mother.

Then Lupe sees the mother's age and sees a possible reason, though not an excuse, for her poor choices. Though she now has four children to care for, the mother of these twins turned eighteen only yesterday. She must have been fourteen when she got pregnant with her first. When she had called the unit to check on her sons earlier, her only response to nurse Jody King's deliberately blunt rundown of the twins' dire condition had been to ask, "Do they have toys?"

"Well, no," Jody had said, baffled. "Your babies can't really move, breathe on their own or open their eyes. They are sedated and on potent painkillers. They almost died. They're very, very fragile."

"Oh," their mother had responded. "Does that mean they can't come home with me tomorrow?"

Jody recounts this conversation for Lupe and suggests that the neonatologist is going to have her hands full with this mother as much as with her babies. Lupe asks why.

"Because," Jody says, "the only other thing she asked was, 'What does 'fragile' mean?'"

The second twin is now on full life support, on very high ventilator settings, with a very dim prognosis. In such cases, the neonatologists seek out the parents, explain everything that has happened, explain that if the baby survives, his life will likely be painful, unfulfilling and short. Then they pose a choice: Do you want us to do everything we can or back off and let nature take its course? Lupe knows she can keep this child alive. She also knows that not one doctor in the NICU would hesitate if the parents said, back off, let him die in peace.

But Lupe finds that the mother cannot, or will not, comprehend the circumstances, leaving Lupe no option but to continue all efforts.

In the old days, doctors alone made these sorts of decisions with parents having little or no say. Doctors were God. Parents were cruelly excluded: They were told what to do, where to sign, and they did it. In the seventies and eighties, this began to change. Medical ethicists advocated a partnership between parents and doctors in such decisions through "informed consent," even if this sometimes made the process infinitely more painful and difficult. Then the government weighed in with misguided rules pushed through by President Reagan in 1984, the so-called Baby Doe Regulations, inspired by one of the president's typically garbled anecdotes, this one about the death of a seriously ill newborn with Down Syndrome whose parents had refused to consent to lifesaving treatment. The president turned a very difficult situation with no easy solution into a simple matter of black and white, right and wrong. The new regulations threatened hospitals with loss of funding and doctors with criminal penalties if they failed to preserve the lives of all babies, even severely damaged ones, unless treatment would be futile. This left many physicians skittish about holding back treatment even in obviously terminal cases, no matter what the parents wanted. But the law was so vague and badly written that no hospital, lawyer, court or physician read it exactly the same way, and the result has been that over time it gradually fell to hospitals, doctors and parents to work out their own solutions to such awful situations, case by difficult case.

In talking to the twins' mother, Lupe uses the words death, dying, critical condition, developmental disability, brain damage. It doesn't matter. The mother keeps asking about toys and when her babies can come home, and saying how she knows everything will be just fine. Lupe says, "Well, would you like me to call a priest?" She knows that often gets parents' attention when all else fails, but not this time. The mother seems bewildered. She asks, "Why?"

In the end, Lupe cannot get a coherent answer from the mother on how to care for the sicker of her twins. Which means she must do everything she can, against her better judgment. The child will live, but Lupe has a sickening feeling that, in the end, no one will be calling his case a miracle.

Then there is Elias Allman. On a night in which every baby in the unit seems to be acting up, as Lupe puts it, Elias decides to go to the top of the list.

"I don't know what to do about Allman," Valerie Josephson tells her a short time later, referring to the baby by his last name, as is customary in the NICU. She's come in from Room 276 to get Lupe's opinion. "He's desatting. He never did that before, not like this. His pH is down. I gave him bicarb."

Valerie sounds disturbed. Sodium bicarbonate, in addition to being a code drug, is given in smaller doses to counteract imbalances in the body chemistry that make the blood too acidic. But such imbalances are only a symptom of a greater problem; if Elias needs bicarb, something else is wrong with him, something no one has yet detected.

"He may be getting septic," Lupe says, looking up from the dinner plate on the desk, a congealed burrito, untouched and cold. "Let's get a culture, CBC. He's off antibiotics—better restart him, gent and vanco. And if he's that bad, we'd better think about moving him back into 288."

When the CBC—the complete blood count—comes back, this quick inventory of white and red blood cells, platelets and various other blood components shows numerous "bands," markers that suggest infection. This is not solid proof of an infection—a culture is needed for that, actually growing a microscopic crop of the disease organism in a petri dish. But that can take twenty-four hours and as long as seventy-two for certain slow-growing microbes, and in the NICU, three days is an eternity, more than enough time for a small infection to become overwhelming inside a preemie whose immune system barely functions and who is using all his reserves of energy just to breathe. A neonatologist never waits for culture results to confirm an infection in a preemie: Broad-spectrum IV antibiotics, gentamicin and vancomycin in Elias's case, are started immediately after the suspicious CBC results come back. This is routine; indeed, even simple rule-out sepsis cases are given antibiotics the minute they enter the unit. There is a consequence of this lavish use of antibiotics, however: the "ecology" of the NICU has become so dominated by drug-resistant bacteria that some of the best antibiotics in the medical arsenal are no longer effective. Hospitals in general and NICUs in particular are inadvertent laboratories for the process of evolution and natural selection—you couldn't design an environment better at breeding drug-resistant bugs. Which is why hand-washing rules are so rigorously policed and the doctors and nurses have the driest, roughest hands around—hygiene lapses can create an epidemic. For Elias, Lupe prescribed the second tier of antibiotics used in the NICU; the drugs must be constantly rotated because germs that are resistant to at least some of the commonly used antibiotics are always present.

But Elias's problems are not simply a matter of infection. Lupe fears other, more immediate problems: His blood gases are bad, his stomach is more of a mess than ever. He still hasn't had a bowel movement—it's been six days now. He has a repogle—a tube that goes through his nose and down to his stomach, designed to relieve built-up gas—but it is not helping his bloat. Yet his X ray shows nothing new. No NEC, no obvious obstruction. Lupe comes back from the X-ray room in the basement shaking her head. It makes no sense.

"There must be something there," she says as she pores over Elias's chart. "But what is it?"

Lupe returns to her cold dinner in the coordinator's office, still looking through Elias's latest labs, while Valerie Josephson races off to a C-section of a thirty-six-weeker, hoping she won't have to admit another baby into the already chaotic NICU population. The resident gets to the OR and finds Mom smiling on the operating table. Dad happily video-tapes the proceedings amid the smell of cauterized flesh as the OB makes his incision and seals off the bleeders—a jarring set of images the young resident tries to ignore. She grabs a blue receiving blanket as her nurse sets up in the corner, and a few minutes later, the dad is leaning in with his camera, saying, "There she is," and Valerie is handed the baby.

The infant flails and cries loudly as the resident strides to the corner and places her on the warmer. The nurse wipes her off and puts an-tibacterial drops in her eyes. The RT suctions her mouth and throat—all clear. The neonatal crew is as precise and efficient as a drill team. The baby is pink, crying, apparently healthy. Seven pounds, eight ounces—a giant compared to most of the NICU customers. The nurse calls out the weight for the parents to hear. The baby pees heartily, always a good sign, as Valerie calls her initial Apgar: nine out of ten. "She looks great, a very healthy girl," Valerie calls to the mom. Dad swings his video cam-era up at Valerie, then back to the baby. Valerie tries to imagine the child being old enough to watch her own birth by cesarean section and can't do it. *I'm* still not old enough for that, she thinks to herself, sup-pressing a smile.

Then the girl grunts a bit, and her nostrils flare. The nurse and Valerie exchange looks, a silent uh-oh. This is a bad sign. Flaring nos-trils and grunting are the first hint of possible respiratory difficulties. The baby may be working harder to breathe than she should. Or it could just be a random expression, a facial tic, a funny cry—meaning-less. The difference is an admission to the NICU for three days or more, or a trip to the newborn nursery, then home tomorrow. The difference is a happy ending for Dad's video or a crushing, scary disappointment.

Val rubs the side of the baby's chin, a way of stimulating her slightly. The baby cries louder; the grunting and flaring stop. She still looks good. Her heart sounds strong and her lungs clear through Valerie's stethoscope.

She's borderline, Val decides. On a slow day, she'd take her to the NICU. But this is not a slow day. She tells the nurse to send her to the transitional newborn nursery. They'll monitor her there, with a pulse oximeter to keep tabs on her oxygen saturation. If there's a problem, they'll call for an NICU admission then. She explains this to the parents, tells them she thinks the child will be fine, then returns to the unit. Lupe gives her the thumbs-up when she sees no new baby in tow. (The newborn nursery keeps her. Valerie made the right call; the baby shows no other symptoms.)

"Finally, we get a break," Lupe says.

Then they start night rounds together, going from baby to baby, trying to figure out who is going to keep them awake tonight. Lupe predicts she'll get two hours' sleep at the most. (She gets one.) Elias and Eric Lee top the list of potential sleep bandits, followed by Nikkol Hawkshaw, who is being suctioned again but is still off the vent, Lupe sees with satisfaction.

"How'd you manage that?" Valerie asks. "I thought she'd never get off."

"I told her I'd sing for her if she didn't get off the vent."

By the time Amalia and Robert arrive a short time later for their usual late-night visit, their son is being wheeled back into Room 288, his graduation to the step-down room abruptly canceled. Karin Nakamura had called to warn them about this, but Amalia still bursts into tears at the sight of her son, sicker than ever.

They watch helplessly as a respiratory therapist hand-bags Elias during the transfer, his oxygen saturation dipped precipitously from the slight jostling during the move. Lupe, Valerie and Karin are all working over him at once, starting new IVs, suctioning his throat and lungs. A huge glob of mucus is removed from Elias's nose, and Amalia looks ready to pass out at the sight. She rushes from the room in tears, one hand covering her face, her voice a husky whisper as she apologizes, "I can't watch this." Robert trails after her, stricken. They had allowed themselves to feel that a corner had been turned after the Roto-Rooter and the move to the step-down room. They feel blindsided. The NICU roller-coaster ride has claimed two more victims.

Lupe, normally attuned to parents in distress, has eyes only for Elias right now. The room is filled with activity, with nurses and RTs attending to several other problematic kids setting off alarms. Lupe briefly glances over at Nikkol Hawkshaw, the gastroschisis patient with the worst jaundice she's ever seen, and instantly regrets it, for she has to try to tune out the awed comment made by the nurse suctioning Nikkol in order to keep her off the ventilator: "My God, look at this poor kid. Even her tears are yellow."

Yellow tears. She's going to have to do something more with Baby Girl Hawkshaw tonight, too. She just hopes it isn't putting her back on the ventilator. Maybe talk to the GI docs about a liver transplant. They have pooh-poohed the notion in the past, but there's not much else to try. She hates the idea of transferring a kid out who hasn't been helped here—Miller does not do infant liver transplant surgery—but if that's what it takes, that's what they'll do. She adds this to her mental checklist, then returns her full attention to Elias. She probes his abdomen yet again. There is something new here, something disturbing: Her gentle squeeze reveals a swollen gut that feels hard to her touch. The skin is darkened, a sign of poor circulation. This is an ominous finding. Elias has indeed turned a corner: the wrong corner.

"I need a new obstructive series as soon as we're done," she tells Karin. The nurse hears that special calmness in Lupe's voice and realizes in an instant that Elias is in trouble. "And I need to get Dr. Kanchanapoom on the phone. Right away."

When the Allmans come back a few minutes later, the activity around Elias has slowed. He appears stable and comfortable, his sats back in the high nineties, his expression peaceful. Karin explains to the Allmans that they need to do more X rays and tests on Elias to figure out what's wrong with his abdomen, and that the surgeon who did the Roto-Rooter is going to check on him later. "It's going to take a while," she tells them.

The Allmans look exhausted and spent. It's well after ten o'clock. Their visit is in tatters; they can't even get close to Elias. Amalia had been hoping to change a diaper tonight. She has gotten to do only two so far, and this simple task looms large in her mind; it is something that links her and her child in a normal, everyday way. Now that's out of the question. When you find yourself longing for dirty diapers, Amalia thinks, how much worse can it be?

"We're going to go home and get a few hour's sleep," she tells Karin. "Tomorrow's Saturday, we'll be in in the morning. We'll call later to see how things are."

Robert and Amalia coo their good-byes to Elias and leave hand in hand. A minute after they walk out, Lupe comes back from a phone conversation with Dr. Kanchanapoom. The latest report from the radiologist, while not pinpointing a bowel obstruction, says such a blockage in Elias's intestines can no longer be ruled out. Lupe says, "This kid's ready to pop. He needs surgery now. He's going to perf. I know it. Visut's coming in."

Perf—perforate. The word makes Karin shudder, for it is one of the worst things that can happen to a baby in the NICU. Lupe fears that Elias's bowel is so plugged and swollen from unrelieved pressures that it is going to burst. And when the intestines perforate, they flood the system with a host of germs that live safely, even beneficially, in the human gut but that, once unleashed inside a sick and fragile preemie's bloodstream, can easily prove fatal.

"We need to get surgical consent from the parents," Lupe says.

Karin shakes her head and frowns. "They just left."

Lupe's jaw drops. "Left? Left what? The hospital?"

Karin nods, lips pursed. "They didn't know. . . . *I* didn't know."

"All right, just page them. Page them now. We need them back in here," Lupe says, and Karin is running to a phone before the neonatologist even finishes her sentence. "We need consent. Tonight. And then we need to get in there before something bad happens."

27

How many times, Robert Allman thinks, *can we experience the worst day of our lives?*

He is sitting with Amalia on a hard hospital chair, staring vacantly at the walls. They are waiting for word from surgery. It has been almost two hours since Elias went in. Amalia is weeping. She cannot seem to stop. Robert has his arm around her and keeps wondering, *When does it get better?*

The first worst day came out of nowhere, when Amalia went into premature labor. No warning, no reason, they still don't know why it happened. SROM, her chart said: spontaneous rupture of membranes. Cause: Unknown. Robert always thought there was supposed to be a reason when something like that happened, but no one could offer any.

Then there was the day Elias came into the world, again without warning, an even worse day. A week and a half had gone by, Amalia's labor had been halted, she was going strong, they were in for the long haul, everything looked good. Then boom! A day that should have been their happiest, and that tiny bruised baby, Elias Jedi Allman, was suddenly here. "My little warrior," Robert calls him, "our chicken in the incubator"—anything to try to lighten the terror of seeing that sad little child in his plastic box, hooked into so many machines.

And now here was yet another worst day ever: the day they realized, for the first time, just how tenuous a grip their son had on life and how easily they could lose him.

They had gotten home to a blinking answering machine. First it was the nurse, Karin, sounding apologetic, asking them to call as soon as they got in. Then another message, this one from Lupe: "We need you here for tests and to meet with the surgeon at eight in the morning."

Visut Kanchanapoom had come in after eleven. He had tried another Roto-Rooter, then given up, agreeing with Lupe that Elias probably needed surgery—and soon. They would need a special set of X rays, a contrast series, which meant Elias would have to be given a radioactive barium enema so that the problem could be clearly seen, providing a road map for the surgeon.

It was a dreary Saturday morning in early December when Robert and Amalia arrived at the hospital. Two nurses and an RT wheeled Elias down to radiology, where he received the barium, then was mounted like a specimen on an acrylic plate. He was flipped and spun so the opaque white fluid would thoroughly coat his bowels, then the X rays were shot. Elias hated the procedure—his vital signs showed that much. He still couldn't cry because of the ventilator.

Dr. Kanchanapoom came out and explained the results to the Allmans: The barium had gone into the large intestine but had been unable to push beyond the tip of the small intestine. More barium was sent through his stomach, and the resulting X ray confirmed a blockage between the large and small intestines. There was a twist or kink, and it was causing all of Elias's problems.

Then the surgeon offered them a choice: Do the operation now, even though there is a higher risk for babies still on the ventilator, or hold off and wait. Elias might need a colostomy or a gastric tube surgically implanted for feeding if he has the surgery, Kanchanapoom said. But even with all that, holding off on the surgery could pose the higher risk: Elias's bowel might perforate, which could be deadly. If that happened, he would need emergency surgery anyway, and the complications could be greater.

"So there's a choice, but there really is no choice," Amalia had said, and they agreed to the surgery, putting Elias's life in Kanchanapoom's hands.

"Would this have happened if Elias hadn't been premature?" Amalia wanted to know.

Visut nodded. It had nothing to do with his being a preemie; this happened in the womb, early in the pregnancy. A malrotation of the intestine happens every now and then. There is no known cause. Then Visut left for the operating room, and Robert and Amalia began their wait.

But Amalia feels a little bit better now about Elias's premature birth. Drying her tears, she tells Robert that maybe it was nature's way of getting him out so the problem could be fixed as soon as possible.

Meanwhile, Elias's nurse watches as the surgeon deftly opens the baby's abdomen and, piece by piece, removes the sausagelike folds of his large intestine, then his small intestine, until he finally comes to the blocked portion. "There it is," he says softly. "Look at that. Just a half turn." The small stretch of tubular intestine looks as if it had been twisted and pinched by a rubber band; Kanchanapoom gives it a half turn the other way, literally untying the knot, then begins reassembling the puzzle. Along the way, he snips off the appendix; once it is out, a surgeon never puts this organ back in.

"Ooh, that's good, baby, nice and pink," the surgeon says. The nurse is relieved to hear that. Pink bowels are healthy bowels. Had the twist in the intestine been too tight, the blood flow would have been cut off and the oxygen-starved parts would be gray or black. The diseased portion would have had to be cut out and the end reconnected, with Elias getting a temporary colostomy until the intestines healed.

It is an incredible procedure to watch, the nurse later tells Amalia, because the removed bowels look impossibly huge, as if they could never fit back inside the baby—a jigsaw puzzle that must be reinserted exactly as it was removed for everything to function properly.

"How can you make sense out of all that?" the nurse now asks Visut as he wraps up the ninety-minute operation.

"I visualize tying shoelaces," the surgeon answers simply. "To me, it's the same."

When Visut emerges smiling in his surgical garb, Robert and Amalia jump up, the surgeon's expression telling them what they needed to know. Amalia starts crying again. This time, her tears are tears of happiness.

With the drama of Elias Allman's emergency surgery over, attention in Room 288 shifts to Eric Lee's grim battle with kidney failure. What started out as a symptom of other problems—infections, anemia, a compromised immune system—has become the single greatest threat to Eric's life. Dr. Steve Cho, the soft-spoken and imperturbable former NICU fellow who is in charge of Room 288 this week, has tried everything in the neonatologist's arsenal, but Eric continues to slip away.

By the day of Elias's surgery, Eric had not peed in two full days. And this simple failure of a bodily function that everyone takes for granted is having devastating consequences. He cannot purge the toxins that build up hour by hour and are supposed to be flushed out in the urine. The cold and unalterable rules of physics are coming into play, the same physics that causes rivers to overflow and dams to burst when water pressure grows too great. The fluid inside Eric has to go somewhere, so it is accumulating in his tissues: His lungs are drowning, his blood pressure is dropping, his heart is being compressed by tidal forces. The infections that his body cannot fight off are too much for him now, and the sensitive kidneys are the first organs to succumb.

Steve has ordered culture after culture, but the lab has been unable to isolate the specific organism pummeling Eric, although everything else points to a massive infection raging inside him. Along with yeast, the enterococcus microbe is the chief suspect. It normally lives in the intestines harmlessly, but in some cases it can attack its host with overwhelming power. The docs have been throwing all their strongest antibiotics into Eric, but his compromised immune system has no fight left in it. He is losing. Day by day, the relentless fluid buildup continues: seventy-two hours; then ninety-six.

Steve puts a Foley catheter into Eric's bladder, hoping to get things moving, and a few drops do emerge. But the flow quickly dries up. It was just some residual from days before, and nothing else comes out.

"I thought for a minute maybe he was coming back one more time," Donna Prochnow says as she leaves that night. "But now . . ." She looks at the baby and whispers, "Are you going to be here when I come in tomorrow, Eric?"

The next day he is still hanging in but getting worse. Steve has to switch him to the oscillating ventilator to keep his lungs working and pump him full of diuretics in an attempt to force his kidneys to switch back on. He is receiving multiple drugs to boost his flagging blood pressure and to try to restart his kidneys, but after a while he is maxed out; the dosages cannot go any higher. All the doctors and nurses can do then is wait and see. "We hate 'wait and see' here," Lupe says at one point. "But sometimes you have to be willing to admit that there's nothing more you can do. The problem is Mrs. Lee, the desire she has for these babies. You know, we'd all like to think every pregnancy is wanted, but let's face it, they're not. *This* is a *very* wanted pregnancy. That's what makes this so hard for her to accept. And so hard for *us* to accept."

By day five, Eric has become difficult to look at, his weight almost doubled by retained fluids. His ears are like sausages. His fingers and feet are like water balloons. He is given large doses of pain reliever—the morphine derivative fentanyl—but still appears to be in terrible pain. His skin, stretched so tightly, starts to crack and break down. Donna gently slathers him with ointment, trying to soothe him, then glances at the monitors. "See, he likes it," she says. "His sats stayed up. That tells me this is okay."

One of the nurses, Kathy Chao, has gotten close to Lisa Lee and has been talking to her quietly every day about what is happening. Lisa has begun spending nights in the family room now, hoping that one morning Eric "will just wake up." Kathy gently tells her that is not likely to happen. And gradually the mother begins to ask different questions. "Are we doing too much?" she asks Kathy one morning, and the nurse has to answer honestly, "I don't know."

That night, around midnight, Jose Perez, during his turn on call, sees Mrs. Lee walking in. "How are you coping?" he asks. And for once the stoic, uncomplaining woman is ready to talk. She *needs* to talk. She tells Jose about her older sister, her handicap, the braces she had to wear in China during their childhood, and how Lisa Lee had outtoughed all the kids who were cruel to her sister. But she also came to know what it is to be handicapped, how hard it has been for her sister. "And I don't want that for my son. What if Eric outlives me and I'm not here to care for him? I couldn't bear that."

Then she asks the question that cuts to the core of things: "How long can he go on without suffering permanent damage?"

"I have to be honest," Jose replies. "I can't answer that. I don't think he's suffering now, I can tell you that, with all the pain drugs we're helping him with. But I do think if things don't improve soon, you will be faced with a decision. If his blood pressure starts to drop, despite all the support we're giving him, then . . ."

Lisa Lee stands up and looks at her three boys. Marlon is now getting very sick, too, starting to look like Eric, swollen, in pain, though he still has a chance. Osmond, on the other hand, has suddenly taken a turn for the better. His infection symptoms are receding, his ventilator settings are down, and he is no longer NPO. He is taking formula by gavage and gaining weight better than anyone else in the room—not edema, but good old-fashioned baby fat. He is beginning to look more like a baby. He is just 30 grams below 1,200, and when he crosses that threshold, he'll be moved to Room 276.

"Go, Osmond!" Meleah Schenk, the social worker, said when she stopped by to see how Lisa was doing earlier that day. Then she gave Lisa a quick hug. "I am so happy for you."

And Lisa smiled for the first time in a long time.

"Some kids just decide to live," Donna Prochnow said happily. "Whether they're supposed to or not."

Lisa walks to Eric's incubator and looks at her child. Room 288 is relatively quiet, the hisses and clicks of life support machinery blending to make a white noise, like waves breaking and frothing on the sand. Eric is the only one of the three she has ever been able to hold. The moment was delicious, but it left her hungry for more.

"Eric was the one who decided it was time to be born," she says finally. "I think he'll decide if it's time to go."

"I agree," Jose says. "Babies do decide."

Elias Allman can't eat for ten days while his bowels heal from the trauma of surgery and the swelling recedes. Even so, he begins to improve dramatically just one day after surgery. He quickly weans from the ventilator—something he couldn't do before his intestines were fixed—and four days after the surgery, Amalia comes home very excited. "I have some great news," she tells Robert. "Tomorrow they plan to extubate Elias! Can you believe it?"

To her chagrin, Robert says, "No, I'm not getting my hopes up. Every time I do, I get disappointed."

And, sure enough, later that night, Karin Nakamura calls to say that Elias has some small bowel loops again. Just gas, nothing to get worried about, she says. But they'll hold off on extubating him until it clears up.

Amalia is terribly disappointed—and a little angry at Robert, as if it were his fault for having so little faith. She knows this is irrational but can't help it. Robert says nothing, and she bites her tongue, avoiding an argument. In truth, they have hardly bickered at all since Elias was born, which Amalia feels is pretty amazing, considering the stress they've been under. Their relationship has come a long way since they lived together years ago and then broke up over what Amalia considered Robert's immature, out-all-night-with-the-boys behavior. They got back together a year later, after Robert courted her for months, unable, he said, to imagine a life without her and very willing to change his lifestyle. They'd been married two years when Elias was born.

The next day, Amalia goes in for her regular early-afternoon visit with Elias. As she is standing at the scrub sink, Jose Perez walks by and asks, "Been in there yet?"

Amalia shakes her head and looks questioningly at the neonatologist, but he just smiles impishly, says, "You'll see," and walks away. Amalia tosses the scrub sponge into the trash and races into the room. She sees, even from across the room, that something is different, but she can't quite tell what it is. Then she reaches Elias's side and sees the sign one of the nurses has taped to the acrylic box: "Look, Ma! No Tubes! Love, Elias." He is off the ventilator.

"Oh, my God!" Amalia squeals. "I can see his face. Look at those cheeks! Big fat Asian cheeks, like they've got balls stuck in them. I can't believe it!" She is grinning and crying and practically dancing a jig in the NICU. He is one month old. His nurse asks, "Wanna hold him?"

"Can I? Really?" Amalia knows there is a twenty-four-hour no-disturb rule for babies just extubated, so they have a chance to stabilize, lowering their risk of having to go back on the vent. "I thought . . ."

"Sometimes you have to forget the rules, it's more important for Mom to hold the baby," the nurse says as she expertly extracts Elias from his incubator, wraps him with a blanket, then hands him to Amalia, who is laughing and crying at the same time.

These are the best moments in the NICU. Patty Rulon appears with a Polaroid camera and starts snapping pictures for Amalia to take home as she exclaims, "I'm so happy for you!"

Amalia has never held her baby before. The expression on her face occupies some place between joy and relief, tinged with a shadow of sadness that it has taken so long to get to this point, to do something she has longed to do since Elias was born. She holds him close, her face touching his, kisses his cheek—another first—and murmurs over and over, "Oh gosh, this is my baby, my baby." Then she suddenly breaks into song, a soft and surprisingly beautiful rendition of "Silent Night."

After a while, Amalia's tears stop and she says, "I thought they decided not to extubate him because of his stomach. Not that I'm complaining or anything, but what happened?"

"Well, Jose was on last night," Elias's nurse says, "and he said, 'I want him off the ventilator. He can have a big tummy extubated.' And so he came off, and he's staying off. He's doing great."

Then the nurse looks at Elias with a critical eye. She needs to see if he is tolerating being held or if he is in danger of desatting. After a moment she smiles. "You know, that's the pinkest he's been all day," she says. "His color's never been better. That's just good lovin'."

Amalia bursts into tears again at this. "I get to kiss him and love him, I can't believe it."

Across the room, another mother bursts into tears at this moment, too: Lisa Lee. Steve Cho and Jose Perez have just suggested to her that the care being given Eric is now doing more harm than good—that he has, in fact, decided it is time to go. A look of panic steals across her face, quickly followed by resignation and tears. Jose explains that Eric's kidneys are essentially dead and will never work again, and that because of this, his suffering no longer has any point. "I think," he tells her as her eyes well over, "we should begin to withdraw some of the support we're giving him."

Lisa takes a deep breath and agrees. It's time. "I don't want him to suffer . . ." she says, then trails off, choking back a sob.

"You're very brave," Jose says, and Lisa Lee suddenly hugs the neonatologist, reaching up and putting her arms around his neck. She is shaking as she sobs into his shoulder. After a while, Eric's nurse begins to shut off the main IV drips until only his pain medication and nourishment are left.

"We'll watch what happens, and then later we can talk about you holding him," Jose murmurs. "After a while."

He glances across the room then and sees Amalia Allman's glowing, tear-streaked face and the baby in her arms, a combination of moments that captures everything there is to know about the heart and soul of the Baby ER: two mothers overcome with emotion, one for a life about to end, one for a life just beginning.

PART IV

GOING HOME

"Package this one to go."

28

Progress Report:

Allman, BB

Day of Life:. . . . 77

Days in NICU: . 77

Status:. . . . . Infant should be able to be discharged home once he is nippling all feedings and exhibiting steady weight gain.

Dear Elias,

Tonight I got to give you a bath!! I was so excited! You had wet your diaper; very wet. So the nurse suggested we give you a bath instead of her doing it later on. First I shampooed your hair, then sponged your body with soap and water. . . . I was so thrilled. . . . I wish we had a camera to capture the moment. But I'm sure we'll have plenty of special times to take pictures.

Love, Mommy

THE HOLIDAY SEASON IS ALWAYS TOUGH IN THE NICU—TOUGH for the families, the staff, the babies. But this year is a bone crusher.

"To Infinity and Beyond," someone has scrawled across the top of the coordinator's big board, which shows a census of seventy-one babies five days into the New Year. It has been building toward this overload for weeks. The unit is so full that a former storage closet had to be converted to a new wing. Everyone is working brutal hours trying to keep up—double shifts, mandatory overtime, and no days off are the norm. The nurses are miserable, losing time to Christmas shop, time with their families, time to ratchet down the stress. The whole hospital nursing staff is in an uproar, with a full-fledged union drive now official.

Amid this turmoil, the unit saw an unusual number of tragedies.

Eric Lee died in his mother's arms four days after his IVs were withdrawn, when Lisa finally asked that his ventilator be disconnected. As Lisa's sister chanted Buddhist prayers at the baby's side, Eric was removed from the machine and taken over to his mother in the family room for a last embrace.

Two weeks later, Marlon followed in his brother's footsteps with a massive infection, including CMV, cytomegalovirus. CMV is a relatively benign organism that infects 80 percent of the population by adulthood, but that can wreak havoc in anyone with a damaged immune system—preemies in particular. Once again, that awful kidney failure and painful swelling occurred, and the neonatologists were helpless to halt it. And once again, Lisa Lee was forced to sign a DNR, to make the decision to end life support, to hold her second son in her arms as he gasped, squeezed her finger, and passed on.

Each baby was dressed up in fine clothes, new shoes, a cap, and they were given red envelopes of paper money and other bits of paper. Lisa and her family held the boys for twenty-four hours in the family room, a tradition from Lisa Lee's Buddhist upbringing. And then each was cremated, so they could move on to the next life as soon as possible. Lisa comforted herself with the notion that Eric and Marlon had bequeathed their strength to their remaining brother, Osmond, which she felt certain would be enough to carry him through.

And then Osmond, who had been doing so well, who had been ready to leave Room 288, fell ill as well, becoming infected and feverish. He had multiple organisms attacking him, too, including CMV.

Lisa stayed with Osmond constantly, talking to him, cajoling him. "You are my good boy," she would say. "You have to live for your brothers. You can't leave me, too."

Throughout these terrible days, Lisa was seriously ill herself, hemorrhaging large amounts of blood, still not fully recovered from her difficult pregnancy. She had to check into the hospital to receive transfusions and to be evaluated for a hysterectomy. Ultimately, she was spared this surgery. She recovered. And so did Osmond.

Osmond Lee had an edge over his brothers—a small one to be sure, but it was all he needed. He had made it through heart surgery, and so he had better circulation than the others. He had gained some weight, having been able to take more nourishment by mouth than his brothers could. His immune system had developed a bit more; he had more reserves to fight off the infections wracking his body. Most important, he never stopped peeing. His kidneys limped on, and the infections finally receded. Osmond had just enough strength to allow the massive treatments the doctors gave him to have a chance to work. His breathing—almost nonexistent for one terrible week—improved.

Finally, two weeks after Marlon died, Osmond came off the ventilator and moved to Room 276, where he began the long, difficult transition to grower-and-feeder status. There would be many setbacks along the way. He would have a terrible time learning to nipple-feed; his instincts were atrophied, his ability to suck was hampered by a mouth and throat too long molded around a breathing tube. Sara Masur worked with him for weeks. The ophthalmologists would discover just in time that he was about to go blind from his long exposure to oxygen therapy. Osmond's vision was saved, for the most part, through laser surgery. Other tests showed he had suffered some hearing loss, a common micropreemie problem. But he would never return to Room 288, and his progress would continue, slow and steady. Donna Prochnow had been right, Lisa Lee later observed. *Some kids just decide to live, whether they're supposed to or not.*

"Osmond decided," she would say. "With help from his brothers."

. . .

Stuart and Kristine Hawkshaw, meanwhile, decided to leave the NICU for another hospital, a last-ditch attempt to save their daughter's life. With the new feeding tube a failure, it became clear that the gastrointestinal physicians who were consulting with the NICU were stumped, at least for the moment, by Nikkol's problems. The doctors and nurses of the NICU do not often—or happily—send patients away without having healed them. Indeed, such occasions, rare as they are, gall them. But if the choice lies between wounded pride and seeking the best possible course of action for a sick infant, nurse Nancy Burkey told the Hawkshaws, there really is no choice. So, with Nancy's encouragement and Art Strauss's support, the Hawkshaws sought help from new gastrointestinal specialists, ones who are part of a program at the University of California–Los Angeles that has helped pioneer liver and bowel transplant surgery, one of only four medical centers in the nation performing such operations on infants. The surgery is very high risk, but Kristine and Stuart Hawkshaw seized on it as their daughter's last, best hope.

"She's made it this far," Kristine told Nancy as they wheeled her to a waiting ambulance. "She'll make it all the way."

The next time Nancy sees the Hawkshaws, it is a few weeks later, on a rolling hill overlooking the ocean at Palos Verde, California—a section of a cemetery that the undertakers call Baby Land. The tiny graves are decorated with pinwheels, stuffed animals and favorite toys. It is a place of unutterable sadness, the place where Stuart and Kristine Hawkshaw say good-bye to the daughter who had been too sick and too damaged for the transplant surgery to work.

Just a few days after Marlon Lee's death, David Rios, who had been making slow progress after many setbacks, crashes at sunrise and must be rushed back to Room 288. David is an old-timer in the unit, and his chart is a veritable medical encyclopedia. He has received at least forty-two separate drugs, every sort of antibiotic, numerous transfusions, IV nutrition—virtually the entire NICU pharmacology. He has had surgeries on his anus—which was closed at birth—his colon (he has a colostomy) and his elbow for an infectious growth eating at the bone. He has been stuck with needles close to a thousand times in his eighty-nine days in the NICU. He has had every test the hospital could offer, from computerized axial tomography (CAT) scan to magnetic resonance imaging (MRI) and every sort of X ray, ultrasound and echocardiogram. The MRI, a long, difficult test in a sealed chamber in a separate building because of the powerful and disruptive magnetic fields inside, was, in a way, a treat for David: Being rolled out of the unit, past the labor delivery department, down the elevator and out into the winter sunshine was his first trip outdoors, except for his ambulance ride from a community hospital the day he was born.

David's diagnosis could not be made for more than a month, when the doctors concluded he had a rare congenital malady called VACTERL, an acronym for the various defects, each of them requiring corrective surgery, that afflict children with the disease: defects of the heart, the lungs, the spine and other areas of the body. But he had to be stable before those surgeries could be attempted, and David was nowhere near stable. He was, as Patty Rulon called him, a train wreck of a kid. His principal problem was a hypoplastic lung—one was shrunken while the other, forced to do all the work, was badly damaged and giving out after months on the ventilator.

Recently he had been doing better, weaned slightly from the vent. He was in a real crib, not an incubator, in Room 276, where he had become a favorite with the nurses, particularly his primary nurse, Susan Gadwa, who talked and visited with him and his mother whenever possible. He had toys he loved, a music box he listened to, pictures he loved to look at. He knew Susan and smiled shyly at her at times; when his mother came in, even on bad days, his vitals would improve and he would calm down. Over the months, he had stopped being BB Rios and had become simply David. Professional detachment fades with long-timers like him. Everyone in the unit knew him, liked him and tried not to think about the fact that his recovery was iffy at best.

Now he has crashed because of yet another massive infection—his fourth such bout. This time, his oxygen saturation plummeted to ten, one tenth of normal. Kim Wibben, his respiratory therapist, bagged him for hours before she finally got him back up to stay. He needed six doses of epi and a shot of the even more powerful heart stimulant atropine. Even then, his ventilator had to be set at record-breaking high pressures just to keep him from crashing again. His sats are still poor, his carbon dioxide levels impossibly high, his heart erratic, his blood pressure dropping. He is dying.

He is loaded with so many pain relievers he ought to be unconscious, but he's not. He's looking around, staring at the doctors and nurses, looking for a familiar face. Lupe cannot believe it. Kim Wibben leans close to him and says, "David, if you're ready to go, you just go ahead." And right on cue, his sats drop again, from the eighties to the twenties. Kim and Susan Gadwa exchange glances. "He's telling us something," Susan says.

Kim, normally unflappable, stifles a sob. She has become very attached to this baby, whose lungs required constant attention from the RTs. She says, "I hope his parents listen to him."

The NICU staff does not pull punches with the parents. They cannot afford to: Parents need to know how sick their children are; otherwise, they are blindsided when things turn out badly. The Rios family was told repeatedly that David's prognosis was poor, that his one working lung could give out at any time, that his stay in the hospital would be long and difficult. The nurses knew how bad he was when he was just a few weeks old; that's why they were talking about DNRs long ago, much to Art Strauss's consternation.

But the Rios family would not or could not accept David's dire condition. From his first days in the unit, they would look at his angelic face, his wispy light hair, his alert, intelligent expression—when it wasn't clouded by pain, which was all too often—and saw only a future in which they brought him home and nursed him to health and a full and happy life. "Isn't that what we're supposed to want?" his mother asked once, and who could say no to that?

She desperately wants him to make it; she is thirty years old, and this is her first child, conceived after years of trying. It has been easy for her to ignore the bad news; she speaks only Spanish, relying on her husband for translation. But if he was told David was doing poorly, he would turn to his wife and say in Spanish, "He's getting better." Not that correcting this helped. When a Spanish-speaking member of the staff overheard the mistranslation and gave her accurate information, the mother just shook her head and said it wasn't true or it didn't matter. She knew David would pull through.

Now, summoned to Room 288, she sees her son's gray pallor and the tight expressions on the faces around him. And no translation is necessary: She understands for the first time that her David will not be coming home. Lupe, who has been working on him for hours with Kim and Susan at her side, explains how David's body has been overwhelmed by infection, how his heart and lungs have been failing even while he has been on tremendous levels of life support. Now there's nothing else to be done, she says. It's time to think about easing David's pain. It's time to think about letting him go.

At these words, Mrs. Rios runs screaming from the room and locks herself in the family room. Her husband, suddenly angry at the doctors, the nurses, the hospital, the world, stalks out after her. Lupe chases after them as the loudspeaker crackles to life in the hushed room, making everyone wince. "Do you want the priest for Rios?" the secretary wants to know.

"No," Lupe answers as she's leaving. "I'd rather he be with the family."

Another RT asks Kim if she would like to take a break. She's been bagging David for so long her arm and hand must be numb. But she says, "No. I *want* to do it." Then she bends and kisses his forehead, stroking him. Susan does the same. "You are such a fighter, aren't you?"

Kim says in a rueful sort of way. "You just ran out of steam." David's eyes are closed now.

After a few moments, Mrs. Rios returns to the room, crying but calmer, her husband at her side, face drained of color. Meleah Schenk, David's social worker, found Mrs. Rios curled on the floor of the family room in a fetal position. "Mrs. Rios," she had said simply, "David needs you now. You should be the one touching him and holding him, not other people." After a moment, Mrs. Rios had sat up. Yes, she said. You're right.

With David's mother in front of his crib in a chair, Lupe speaks quietly with her and her husband. They both nod after a while, and Lupe takes the breathing tube from David's mouth and puts him in his mother's arms. Mrs. Rios covers her baby with kisses. Tears are streaming down Kim's and Susan's faces. Later, they will criticize themselves for not being professional, for not staying detached. But they cannot help it: They love this little boy.

Two other nurses draw privacy screens around David and his parents. Elsewhere in the big room, diapers are being changed, parents are cooing at their children, nurses are chatting, the loudspeaker comes alive again, summoning people to case management rounds in the coordinator's office—the busy world of the NICU spins on.

Without the machines and drugs and tireless efforts of RTs, doctors and nurses, David's heart rate drops from just above a hundred beats per minute to the seventies, then the sixties, then the thirties. He hasn't opened his eyes in a while—everyone assumes he is gone already, even though his body is still nominally functioning. But then those big gray eyes flutter and look up at his mother, just a flicker. Then he closes them. A few moments later, there is a flat line on the heart monitor. After another minute or two, Lupe gently takes him back. The parents stagger from the room as Lupe listens for a heartbeat with her stethoscope. There is none. She notes the time for the record: "I'm calling it 10:08." There is nothing else for her to say or do. She looks at the stricken faces around her, then slowly walks over to a new admission, a tiny four-hundred-gram baby born within the hour. "Okay," she sighs, "what've we got here?"

Susan has one more job to do for David, however. She gently disconnects him from his wires and IVs, then carries him back to the treatment room. She shuts the door and puts him on a table, where she washes and dresses him, musing over how hard it is to accept that they cannot help everyone in the NICU.

Susan takes his picture and puts his footprints on a card, speaking softly and lovingly to her patient as she works. She is constructing a "bereavement package" for the parents. It sounds awful, macabre, Susan says, but the parents appreciate it later. David looks better in the instant snapshot than he has ever looked before.

"I have seen a lot of things while working here," Susan muses in the quiet room. "And you tend to get spiritual over time. It comes with the territory. For me, it's reincarnation: I have come to believe that babies choose their parents, and they choose what body they'll have. And sometimes I look at these kids and say, 'Why did you pick *that* body?' David picked a really tough, tough body. For some reason, he needed that experience. But after three months of getting stuck, suffering, having so much wrong with him, having so much pain, he was ready to find another body. I hope he's easier on himself the next time around."

And then Susan takes David back to his parents. They will spend as long as they need with him in the family room—minutes, hours, whatever they wish—saying good-bye. Then Susan will fulfill her last duty to David: She will bundle him up tightly and carry him, gently, kindly, slowly, on the long walk downstairs.

29

"LET'S PACKAGE THIS ONE TO GO," LUPE TELLS A MED STUDENT A FEW days later. She is working the Fat Farm now, the last stop in the NICU before discharge. The med student looks at her blankly.

Lupe groans. "Didn't anyone show you how to put together a discharge package?" The student shakes his head. That means Lupe is going to have to do both her student's work and her own today. She sighs. "Okay, lesson one. First you pull the chart . . ."

The mood in the unit has changed abruptly, much to everyone's relief. It is just as crowded and busy as before, still overfull, but the spate of tragedies has quickly been followed by success. Several dramatic codes ended happily. A twenty-four-weeker came through with flying colors, with none of the complications the Lee boys experienced. The newer babies coming in are not so sick—they are healing and leaving faster than their predecessors, with fewer complications. And the older kids, who seemed to linger so long on the intensive list, are finally getting better. Things are back to normal.

Steven Hachigan is the first to go. As David Rios was being handed to his mother, Steven was being set up for a pneumogram—a twenty-four-hour study of his breathing patterns, focusing most intently on when he is asleep. He continues to suffer from absence-of-breathing spells—he remained the King of ABs while in Room 276, a title awarded to only one baby in the unit at any one time—but has slowly gotten better. One of his key medicines now is caffeine, a powerful stimulant of the respiratory center for infants.

The test results show Steven still has some rocky periods in his sleep when he desats—he'll need to go home with a monitor and oxygen tanks. But he should grow out of that in a few months.

Monique and Mark Hachigan are delighted to be taking him home, of course, but they are worried, too. He looks chubby and healthy now, up to five and a half pounds, eating well. But who knows what will happen in the next year? Will he get cerebral palsy, developmental delays? Will his eyes go bad, despite the clean bill of health from the ophthalmologist?

Gnawing at Monique most is the fact that she has come to depend on the nurses in the unit to take care of her baby. The impressive list of medications he'll need, the oxygen, the monitor—all those will now fall largely on her and on the part-time nurse they have hired until things settle down. Monique has had to learn CPR, how to set up oxygen. She is constantly worried about screwing up. "Maybe I'll leave him here till he's potty-trained," she jokes.

"Oh, you'll be fine," Margie Perez assures her. "And *he's* going to be fine."

On the day of discharge, Monique and Mark carry their son out, hauling a big bag of diapers, medicines and his monitor and oxygen. Art Strauss runs into them in the hall. "Well, hello and good-bye," he says. "This is a big step." Then he offers some advice to a bemused Monique: "These kids don't like sensory deprivation after living here. You turn the lights down and keep it quiet, and they go nuts. Better to keep a light on and the music on. It takes a few months for them to rediscover their circadian rhythm."

Mark has turned on a video camera to record the departure. Margie Perez comes out, bubbling with excitement, and waves at the camera: "Hi, Steven, I changed your diapers. He'll see this when he's maybe thirty, this'll be great. You're going home, baby!"

"Do you think he knows he's going home?" Monique asks.

"Oh, he's ready to go," Margie says. "You can always tell. When a baby is crying to be held, wanting to be picked up, fussing all the time—basically driving us crazy—then you know it's time for him to go home. He's ready."

"Ready or not, here we go," Monique says.

Little Ella, the drug baby transported by Julie France during the pre-holiday crush, is next to go, discharged to foster care. After a few bad weeks, her withdrawal symptoms faded as expected, and she began to behave like a normal healthy baby.

Jessica Jones, whose brain was destroyed by cocaine, has not improved, as expected. After many illnesses, none of them life-threatening, she goes to a special medical foster home, where she can receive around-the-clock care. She has a G-tube surgically implanted in her stomach, the only way she can eat. Her mother is petitioning the court for visitation privileges and custody. No legal action has been taken against her for her drug use during pregnancy.

Baby Girl Berger's progress continues to surprise and please everyone in the unit right up until the day she goes home. The little girl who was coded for twelve minutes in the OR, then brought back to life by Lupe, is nippling all her meals. She cries and focuses her eyes and reacts appropriately when touched or tickled. She laughs. Her abysmal prognosis has evaporated; though there are many challenges ahead and she may yet prove to be profoundly affected by her traumatic birth, she has a shot at a life, a real life. Sara Masur calls her a living miracle. Her parents, after many dark days, have learned to smile again.

Jordan Leos is next out the door. The little boy with Down Syndrome and a defective heart has been slow to take to bottle feeding. Down's babies have trouble figuring out where to put their tongue—they stick the nipple underneath, then can't suck—but he finally gets the hang of it after Sara Masur shows Maricela Leos how to pull his chin down and get him to suck correctly. Soon he is drinking his formula with little hesitation. He'll go home and return for heart surgery in seven or eight months.

"I can't wait to have my little angel home," Maricela says as she walks him out the door. "All our prayers have been answered."

Even Osmond Lee is on the march toward recovery, slowly but surely. He leaves the NICU on his 116th day of life, oxygen bottle and monitor in tow, and the only remaining medical problems left—besides his damaged lungs and weak eyesight—are two large hernias. They will be taken care of in outpatient surgery. He looks like a completely different baby from the one in Room 288, up to five pounds, fifteen ounces—a giant compared to his tiny birth weight.

Like the other parents here, Lisa Lee has learned to diaper and bathe and feed her baby in the hospital. She has also grown dependent on the NICU, her and her baby's safety net. Still, though she is fearful of the future, she is looking forward to taking him home and ending her daily two-hour trips to and from the hospital. "When he's home, I'll take the day shift, my sister will take the night shift, we'll be with him all the time," she tells Osmond's primary nurse, Kathy Chao. "Just like here."

As she gathers up all his medicines, his oxygen equipment, his clothes and blankets and toys, she says, "Someday, when he's old enough, I'll tell him about his brothers, and everything he went through here, the heart surgery, the infections, the eye surgery."

"Oh, that's not such a bad list," Kathy says, holding Osmond for the last time. The baby is gurgling happily. "That's all pretty standard stuff here."

Lisa Lee raises an eyebrow. "Standard? Not for the mom. Nothing about any of this is standard for the mom."

And then a very proud mother, with her sister and father in tow, walks out of the hospital with Osmond nestled in a car seat.

The crunch gradually slows down and life assumes a less crazed rhythm in the NICU. The number of babies declines further. The seriousness of their illnesses abates a bit more. The unit can breathe again.

Some other distractions evaporate around the same time. As the shake-up of the medical economy continues unabated, the threats to the NICU in Long Beach and the doctors who run it seem to lessen. The perinatal practice next door is indeed bought by a larger company—the one the NICU doctors hoped for, Magella Healthcare. The company makes a friendly offer to acquire the NICU practice as well, which the Four-Headed Dragon politely declines.

Meanwhile, the rival conglomerate, Pediatrix, which once seemed poised to make a move on the NICU, seems far less a threat. Its stock price tumbled from a high of sixty-four dollars a share to less than nine, and it came under investigation in several states amid allegations of billing irregularities. There are no other threats to the neonatal practice on the horizon other than the usual budget constraints, insurance hassles and other everyday realities of modern medicine. It seems the neonatal practice at Long Beach is secure for the foreseeable future: Doctors Art Strauss, Penny Jacinto, Jose Perez and Lupe Padilla are in for the long haul.

Of course, there are more distractions to fill the void left by the old ones, not the least of which is the appointment of Lupe as chief of staff of the children's hospital—yet another passel of meetings to enter into her electronic organizer. She downplays the honor—"I didn't say no fast enough"—but she is clearly pleased by the new position and the chance it gives her to chart some new courses for the hospital.

The nurses of the NICU have less cause to feel optimistic. They continue to work long hours and difficult shifts, loving the work but sometimes feeling underappreciated by their employer. The entire Long Beach Medical Center nursing staff, including the NICU nurses, eventually holds a union election. It fails by ten votes.

A few weeks before Elias Allman's original due date, his parents give him his evening bath. It's been a wonderful visit. Elias has been moved to an open cradle—no more incubator, no more IVs. Just a little oxygen and his pulse oximeter tether him to the hospital.

They have a good feeding session, too—Elias does his best ever—and he has never seemed more alert, more attuned to their presence, really focused on his mom and dad in a new way. If this keeps up, the nurses say, he'll be able to go home on his due date, just as Patty Rulon predicted so many months earlier. Amalia leans over and says, "We're so proud of you. You did so well today, yes, you did."

She then rocks him to sleep, another first. He just seems to melt against his mother, snoring softly, at peace in this room full of noise and light and conversations. He sleeps soundly through it all, even as a fifteen-year-old mother—who has just given birth to her second child—carries on at the other end of Room 276, complaining about her infant's bili lights, complaining about the ventilator (which the mother thinks exists simply to stifle crying, leading her to exclaim, "I gotta get me one of those to take home!"), complaining about the fact that she has a baby at all. The baby's grandmother is adding to the din, loudly apologizing for her teenage daughter, promising she will take care of this grandchild, as she has done with the first one, so her daughter can go out and party and have fun, "like teenage girls are supposed to do." To which the new mother says, "Damn right. I'm not staying home for no baby. Even with one of these damn no-crying machines." And still Elias sleeps, oblivious.

In its own bizarre way, this is the most natural parental moment the Allmans have ever had. Elias has fallen asleep on *his* time—not because it was part of the NICU schedule but because he was exactly where he wanted to be, nestled in his mother's arms, doing exactly what he wanted to do. Robert comes over, puts his arm around Amalia, and leans down to kiss his son.

"Yes, we are so proud of you, Elias," he murmurs.

· · ·

As Elias's original due date nears, his condition is upgraded by the NICU staff. He is no longer considered acutely ill. He is, officially, a grower and feeder.

His progress has been steady since his surgery, with very few setbacks. He needs only a trickle of oxygen to support his damaged lungs, which are slowly healing. More than half his nourishment is now by bottle and the rest by gavage, and he is also breast-feeding, much to Amalia's delight. When he can take all his nourishment from breast or bottle and the gavage tube is stowed for good, Amalia and Robert are told, he will have reached the milestone of "nippling all feeds." Then he can go home.

This is happening a bit more slowly than his parents would like to see—Elias tires easily when feeding, and he has not adjusted to working for his meals as easily as some. But Sara Masur has had several sessions with him and Amalia and has assuaged the parents' fears that something might be wrong.

"Every baby develops at his own pace," she explained. "Elias needs a little more time. The connections in his brain will happen—they're happening now. Just be patient."

Elias's change in status has had one other important effect: The Allmans' HMO has demanded that his care be transferred to one of its own pediatricians, a doctor who has staff privileges in the NICU but who is there only a few hours a week. Because Elias is no longer acutely ill, the hospital bylaws do not require around-the-clock staffing by his attending physician—he can just leave orders for the nurses to follow. Everything else stays the same for him: the nurses, his location in the unit, Sara's work with him. Just the doctor changes, which saves the HMO money.

But the HMO has a different mandate. The goal of the attendings in the NICU has been to get Elias to accept all his nourishment by bottle or breast before going home, just like a full-term baby. The HMO's goal is to get Elias out of this very expensive NICU as soon as possible.

When Amalia's original due date arrives a few days later and Elias is still not ready to go home, the new doctor suggests that his slow feeding might indicate a neurological problem. He calls in a neurologist to examine Elias for possible brain abnormalities that might be impairing his development.

Amalia and Robert are terrified; no one had ever suggested anything like this before. They knew preemies were at risk for brain bleeds, but all of Elias's head ultrasounds had been unremarkable, and Art, when he wrote up the transfer-of-care report, made a point of saying that Elias's brain and nervous system appeared normal. And the Allmans know their child, they can see how he is coming along, how aware and alert he has become. It just doesn't seem possible to them that he is impaired in some way.

When Sara Masur hears about the impending consult, she is outraged and discouraged. She has been seeing steady and fairly rapid improvement in Elias's nippling, as have the nurses caring for him. From her perspective, his problem is both simple and natural: He simply has not outgrown his preemie way of dealing with too much stress or sensory input—which is simply to go to sleep. When normal babies are overloaded, they fuss and cry; preemies sleep. That's why the myth that preemies can't feel pain persisted so long—instead of wailing, their nervous systems shut down. Sometimes, when feeding, Elias shuts down, though this is happening less and less with each passing day. Two more weeks, maybe three, Sara believes, and he will have outgrown the problem. Then he should be ready to go home.

The Allmans eventually decide that there could be more than one reason their HMO wants a neurological consult. If the neurologist found the smallest suggestion of a brain abnormality, the HMO could seize on that as a justification for surgery to equip Elias with a gastric tube. He could then be force-fed directly through his stomach and be discharged in a matter of days instead of weeks, saving the HMO thousands of dollars in the process while Robert and Amalia tube-feed their baby at home. Never mind that such surgery would pose a severe developmental setback for Elias; it would be economical.

The Allmans prepare for battle, but it is not necessary. To everyone's relief, the neurologist gives Elias a clean bill of health. He doesn't need surgery, she says, all he needs is a little more time.

As it turns out, he needs only two more weeks.

⌒

Dear Elias,

Today is Valentine's Day and it's the best ever. We got to bring you home today!!! It's one of the happiest days of our lives, but I know we will all have many more!

Your dad and I will celebrate your birthday twice. Even though you were born on November 15th (another happy day), your life with us as a family begins today.

Elias, we love you so much. You're our little angel sent from God. We're looking forward to the future and being the best parents we can be.

Love, us both,
Mom and Dad

Epilogue

NEONATOLOGY CONTINUES TO OCCUPY THE CUTTING EDGE OF medicine, saving tiny lives on a daily basis, with revolutionary advances on the horizon in this new century promising to rival those pioneered during the last.

Experimental gene therapies seem to hold the greatest potential at the moment. They represent possible cures for an array of genetic disorders in infants, from the blood disease hemophilia to a rare but crippling immune system disease—popularly known as "bubble-boy syndrome"—that leaves children defenseless against all disease organisms. Gene therapies used on these bubble babies in France have converted their broken immune systems into fully functioning ones, using designer viruses and cells grown in the laboratory to give these children a shot at normal lives. Such therapies hold the promise of someday correcting many other congenital defects seen in the NICU, not only after birth, but from within the womb. Researchers believe even such dreadful diseases as Trisomy 13 could one day be cured with gene therapy if detected and treated during the earliest stages of pregnancy.

Indeed, the most promising advances now seem to lie less in nurturing ever-smaller babies born too soon than in attacking ailments of the newborn *before* birth. In addition to gene therapies, successful surgeries have been performed on fetuses still in the womb that have corrected lung and spine defects—using nature's own life support system to sustain the patient inside the placenta after surgery, rather than the comparatively clumsy devices and technology that man has built as substitutes. Such advances are occurring throughout the world at a breakneck pace, making research into the care and treatment of newborn—and unborn—children one of the most exciting fields of medicine.

But there is a caveat: While such revolutionary treatments for birth defects and genetic anomalies could indeed provide miracle cures for once incurable conditions, they will not address the overarching problem of premature birth itself, in which an otherwise normal child simply enters the world too soon. The mechanism of premature birth is still not well understood—in four out of ten cases, no cause is even identified. So for many preemies, neonatology will remain a game of catch-up.

It is here that those who expected a continuing march of advances in saving and healing ever-smaller premature babies have been disappointed. The same barriers to viability and survival have held fast for more than a decade, and visions of new breakthroughs—of artificial wombs and ventilators that use liquid instead of air, mimicking the conditions *in utero*—have been frustrated by technological limitations and the essential fragility of the human organism before the twenty-fourth week of gestation. Many believe that an absolute limit has been reached, not out of a lack of scientific ingenuity but because of the inherent limitations of the human body. After more than two thousand years, man's scientific genius has managed to shave only four weeks or so from Hippocrates' ancient nostrum about the viability of premature babies, and the prospects of further advances on this front appear unlikely for the immediate future.

At the same time, the problem of premature birth is a growing concern in the United States, where the proportion of babies born before term seems to creep upward with each passing year. New studies tracking the lives of premature babies as they enter school and reach adulthood have lent a depressingly negative cast to this trend: It turns out that people born prematurely in the 1970s and 1980s have suffered lasting disability and impairment in later life in much greater numbers than anticipated. More than half of the smallest preemies tracked by researchers in later life—babies born below 1,500 grams or before thirty-

two weeks—have below-normal intelligence and abnormal brain conditions once they reach school age. Half of the smallest preemies now
entering adulthood required special education programs in school, and
half of micropreemies—those born under 800 grams—are disabled in
some significant way as adults by hearing loss, vision loss, cerebral
palsy, mental retardation or a whole constellation of life-changing im-
pairments. Many of these conditions were not apparent when the babies left the NICU, becoming obvious only as a child entered the
toddler years or school age and important developmental milestones
came slowly or not at all. (On the other hand, the news is not all grim.
Larger preemies fare quite well in the studies: Nine out of ten babies
born after the twenty-eight-week mark remain free of major disabilities
throughout life—only the very small, very early preemies face the high
odds of being disabled.)

Whether the smallest preemies born more recently will fare better
than their predecessors is unknown, although they, too, are being
tracked by researchers, awaiting a verdict. The advent of surfactant
therapy and improved ventilator technology in the 1990s has shortened
NICU stays and greatly reduced the amount of time babies spend on
ventilators, which should mean better outcomes and fewer developmental problems for today's preemies (the general rule being that the
longer the stay in the NICU and on the ventilator, the greater the likelihood of disability and developmental delay in later life). On the other
hand, these same revolutionary treatments have increased the likelihood of survival for the most fragile micropreemies—precisely those
babies who are most susceptible to disability and developmental delay.
Once again, the quicksand nature of neonatology attaches a cost to
every miracle.

The new studies of how preemies fare as they grow up have added a
sense of urgency to efforts under way in many of the nation's NICUs to
provide new types of "developmental" care alongside conventional
medical treatments. The goal is to minimize and compensate for the
pain and other potentially harmful effects that lifesaving intensive care

can have on babies, the hope being that preemies will do better in later life as a result. These efforts range from a redesign of NICU environments to reduce noise and light, to the use of massage, classical music and other therapies to calm infants, to a more generous use of pain-relieving drugs and the relatively simple technique of putting "toaster" covers on incubators to shield the babies from bright lights. Some drugs that have been staples in neonatal units for years are now being reexamined to see if their prolonged use may harm the brain and mental development of preemies.

Concern also continues to mount about the dangers of aggressive fertility treatments and the likelihood they are contributing to the nation's skyrocketing number of multiple births, many of them premature and at risk for illness. Calls for reform have followed several highly publicized multiple births in which some of the infants either died or faced life-threatening ailments. The leading fertility medicine group in the United States, the American Society for Reproductive Medicine, has changed its guidelines to recommend that doctors transfer just two embryos when performing *in vitro* fertilization on women under age thirty-five. If followed, this new policy could greatly reduce the number of multiple births and related prematurity.

The impact of this change remains unclear, however, because the guidelines are voluntary and far from absolute; the organization also endorses the transfer of up to five embryos at a time in certain cases. The practice of implanting large numbers of embryos remains a source of controversy and is banned in some countries in order to limit the risks of premature multiple births and infant deaths. British law, for example, bars the implantation of more than two embryos at a time under any circumstances. No such legal limits exist in the United States, where the lucrative field of fertility medicine is not regulated—each doctor and patient follows his or her own conscience and desire in choosing how many embryos to implant. Fertility doctors in the United States have opposed government regulation because they argue that, unlike British socialized medicine, where even repeated fertility treatments are paid for by the state, Americans must pay for their own. Therefore, it is argued, patients anxious to bear children should be able to maximize the chance of success with a single treatment by having a greater number of embryos implanted, even if this increases the risk of multiple, premature births and illness. Many neonatologists object to this reasoning, which they believe puts money before safety, but there are no further reforms on the horizon.

Parents of preemies, meanwhile, are beginning to demand more information about their choices and consequences in neonatal care. The Internet is alive with discussion groups and Web sites that link parents and former preemies who have survived the NICU, and a difficult and emotional debate is taking shape over when lifesaving treatment should be provided and when it should be withheld. Some parents of profoundly disabled preemies, whose lives have been forever altered by the constant care they must provide their children, complain that they never understood what they were buying into when they consented to heroic efforts to save their tiny, damaged infant. They want more information and more decision-making power when it comes to life-and-death matters in NICU care, so that future preemie parents know what they are getting into—and are empowered to say no when it is clear that a lifetime of profound disability is the likely consequence of their infant's survival. Other parents are equally adamant that heroic efforts must always be made to save babies, even when grave disability is likely—because there is no way to know for sure how things will turn out and because their children, no matter how damaged, still give them great joy.

A resolution of these questions remains elusive, and they are a frequent source of discussion and soul-searching among the neonatologists in Long Beach. They believe strongly in making parents their partners in such important decisions, a position endorsed by the American Academy of Pediatrics but applied with varying degrees of success around the nation. Policies can only go so far in any case, as the neonatologists all too often find themselves handcuffed by pressures beyond their control. Decisions must be made in a split second, sometimes with a dearth of medical information, when they are summoned on a moment's notice to a crash C-section and an infant in distress—emergency situations with little time for talk and no time for reflection. They often are greeted by parents who are under enormous stress or in a state of denial, and who did nothing to educate themselves in advance about the complications and difficulties of premature birth during their pregnancy because they never thought it could happen to them.

And so neonatologists and parents who find themselves thrown together by biology and fate, by the hopes and dreams attached to every new life entering this world and the desperation we feel when those dreams are threatened, almost always prefer to err in favor of doing everything possible. The consequences of this, good and bad, must be set aside for later. In the end, this is not a scientific question. It is not a question to be decided by statistics or ultrasounds or Apgar scores. It is a question of the heart. In the end, there is no real choice in the face of the unknown: We do what we can to preserve life, and hope for the best. The alternative, after all, is no hope at all.

For some parents, questions are all that remain once they leave the NICU. A year after their daughter's death, Stuart and Kristine Hawkshaw still ask themselves if they did too much or too little for Nikkol, whose tortuous seven-month life in the hospital ended when her liver transplant surgery failed mere moments after it began.

They visit her small grave once a week at the hilltop of Baby Land, bringing flowers and toys like so many other parents who come to this place, looking and longing. It's Kris, mostly, who insists on this regular pilgrimage, adamant about maintaining a relationship denied them when their Nikky still lived.

After losing their daughter, the Hawkshaws felt more than grief. Grief was expected. What they didn't anticipate was feeling as if their lives had been stripped of all purpose. Their existence for so long had revolved around sickness and frustration and daily visits to the hospital, they had forgotten what life had been like before. For so long, it had been all they talked about, all they thought about, all they did, and when the dread and the hope and the vigils at Nikkol's side were gone, their days seemed to stretch out before them, hollow and pointless. There was nothing left to fight for, nothing, even, to fight about. They would come home from work and sit and stare at each other, not knowing what to say or do.

Had it not been for Stuart's son and daughter from his first marriage and their innocent insistence that he and Kris return to doing all the things they had been missing for so long—the hikes and ball games and board games and Cub Scout trips—the Hawkshaws might not have survived as a couple. Many parents in their situation do not. But the kids eased them back from the brink. At first it was stiff, a mere going through the motions. Gradually, though, they found their way to normalcy again, or something close to it, to beach outings and surfing and dancing and recognizing just how important these moments were— how irreplaceable and vulnerable and quickly gone the times with our children are. "That was Nikkol's gift to us," Stuart says now. "She reminds us, every day, how precious our children are to us and what a shame it would be to miss even a minute of time with them. Most people have no idea how lucky they are."

After a few months, Kris learned she was pregnant. A year after Nikkol's death, Kelley Hawkshaw, a healthy, perfect, nine-pound boy, was born. Kelley's arrival couldn't have been more different than Nikkol's: He came home from the hospital in a day. And on sunny, perfect afternoons, on a windswept hill dotted with pinwheels and teddy bears overlooking the cool gray Pacific, Kelley Hawkshaw visits his sister.

While the Hawkshaws healed and found new purpose, Jordan Leos had two successful surgeries for his heart defect, and at seventeen months, he is a sweet and gentle addition to the Leos family, doted on by his older brother and sister.

As expected, his Down's Syndrome has slowed—but by no means stopped—his growth and development. He is using a baby walker to motor around the house, usually at high speeds, and is nearly close to walking independently. He is beginning to talk, and he already understands many words. His progress has encouraged both his doctors and his parents, Enrique and Maricela, who feel he will prove to be on the higher-functioning end of the Down's spectrum.

And Enrique Leos is still looking forward to someday driving a school bus with his son on board.

Osmond Lee, the lone survivor of twenty-four-week triplets, enjoyed one glorious month at home with his mother, feeding well, growing well, making steady progress. Then, despite antiviral injections, he contracted a respiratory virus that worsened much more quickly than his new pediatrician anticipated. Such infections can be serious in any small baby, but they pose a particularly grave risk for the damaged lungs and overtaxed immune systems of micropreemies like Osmond.

In the middle of the night, Osmond went into respiratory arrest. Lisa Lee and her sister attempted CPR and called paramedics, but by the time he was revived, Osmond had suffered terrible brain damage. He has been on a ventilator ever since, breathing through a tracheotomy, eating through a gastric tube. His brain appears to have stopped growing, a condition called microcephaly. He requires round-the-clock care at a facility near Lisa's home in La Verne, California, and may never come home. Now, once again, Lisa Lee is being urged to sign a DNR for her sole surviving son, just as she did for each of his brothers. She is being told, once again, that treatment will do more harm than good.

This time, this option appears to be unbearable to Lisa. She knows the outlook is not good for her son, but she is still seeking other medical opinions and may turn to nontraditional therapies, such as acupuncture, to see if something, anything, might help Osmond find his way back to life. "I am not ready to give up on Osmond," she says. "And he is not ready to give up either."

. . .

Little Steven Hachigan did well after leaving the hospital, quickly dispensing with his oxygen and respiratory monitor and growing rapidly, a cuddly, wavy-haired child with a big smile.

The Hachigans had a nurse helping them at home for a week after Steven's discharge, but then Monique felt she was ready to take on the care of her fragile new son on her own. The experience of having Steven in the NICU and caring for him seems to have helped her find a new strength and confidence. The inevitable setbacks preemies must endure—the repeated ear infections and other ailments that have made Steven a regular at his pediatrician's office—have been taken in stride.

When Steven was seven months old, however, Mark and Monique got some bad news: It appeared that all those bouts of apnea and breathing difficulties in the NICU, in which Steven's oxygen saturation levels plummeted, had collectively taken their toll on his brain. He has a form of cerebral palsy called spastic triplegia that was not apparent until he got older. The "motor strip" area of his brain was damaged by oxygen deprivation, and it affects his ability to walk, sit up and use his left hand. His limbs all function, but he moves three of them awkwardly; his left hand moves clumsily, jerkily, as if it were asleep. At eighteen months, he is still struggling to sit up unsupported when playing with his toys, a source of occasional frustration for him and heartbreak for his parents.

At one time in her life, Monique might have gone to pieces over this, she says. Now, though she did cry herself to sleep the night she and her husband learned Steven's diagnosis, she got up the next day and helped her son with his new regimen of exercises designed to stretch and strengthen his weakened muscles. He goes to occupational and physical therapy three times a week with her and is making progress.

The good news is that a child's brain growth during his first three years is tremendous and rapid, which means there is an excellent chance that new neural connections can be forged to bypass the damaged motor strip and let him move more easily and fluidly. Meanwhile, his right hand works fine. And he remains a happy, intelligent boy, learning words and showing no apparent damage to other parts of his brain.

"It will come slowly for him," Monique says with confident firmness. "But it will come. He's going to be okay."

Elias Jedi Allman is a big boy now; the oxygen and monitor that came home with him are long gone. At first, every whimper, cry or cough was a source of fear for Amalia and Robert, so conditioned were they to expect the worst. It took time, but gradually they relaxed, normal parental concerns slowly taking the place of post-NICU paranoia.

Anyone can see that Elias is right where he should be in terms of size and development—if you correct his actual age by the three months he missed in the womb. At fifteen months old, he looked and acted like a one-year-old, which is just as it should be for an otherwise healthy premature baby. "Age adjustment," the parents of preemies call it: He walked and talked three months later than most full-term babies, but other than that, he is a healthy, smiling toddler with no medical issues and two parents who are finding it increasingly hard to remember the details of those frightening three months in the NICU.

These days, only the best moments still stand out in sharp relief: the first time each of them held Elias, the first time they bathed him. The day they brought him home.

Robert and Amalia had talked many times about what they would do that first day they brought Elias to their apartment. When they finally got the chance, they took him into the bedroom and lay down on the bed, and Robert said, "Elias, this is your home, and this is where your life with your family begins. So today is like your birthday for us. You're going to have two birthdays."

When Elias was fourteen months old, there was yet another birthday to celebrate in the Allman household: a little brother's. Joshua Lucas Allman, eight and a half pounds and right on time, joined the family without a hitch. There was no emergency, no trip to the NICU, no neonatal team summoned to the delivery room, no stress beyond that of a normal infant delivery—which, though enormous for most couples, seemed almost anticlimactic for Robert and Amalia.

"It was pretty boring," she observed later in the blasé manner only a graduate of the Baby ER can manage. "The nurses couldn't believe it when I said it seemed easy. But it did."

Resources

The following organizations and Internet sites provide a sampling of some of the information available to parents and others about premature and ill newborns, neonatology, and related issues. There are many other sources of information and support available through local hospitals, medical associations and charitable organizations.

General Premature Baby Information

EdwardHumes.com: The Baby ER section of the author's Web site contains useful links about prematurity and various resources for parents, as well as updates of this resource list and other subjects raised in this book: http://www.edwardhumes.com

For Parents of Preemies: Excellent introduction to the medical, physical and emotional challenges facing premature babies during and after their stay in the NICU, produced by the University of Wisconsin and The Center for Perinatal Care at Meriter Hospital, Madison, Wisconsin. Available in book form for $10 or free on the Internet. Meriter Hospital, Neonatology 6C, 202 South Park Street, Madison, WI 53715. World Wide Web:
http://www2.medsch.wisc.edu/childrenshosp/parents_of_preemies/

Preemie-L: A very complete and informative Web site for parents with children born six weeks or more early, and their family and friends. The site provides links to several excellent e-mail discussion groups. A separate e-mail group for parents of older former preemies is also accessible here, along with extensive fact sheets on the various health problems preemies can face and answers to frequently asked questions. Internet only: http://www.preemie-l.org

Comeunity: Premature baby–Premature child: Maintained by pree-mie parents Rick and Allison Martin, this Web site provides an exten-sive collection of articles, resources and information from doctors, researchers and parents on all subjects related to prematurity, the spe-cial needs of children, coping with prematurity in the family, and what to expect not only in the immediate aftermath of premature birth but also in the months and years that follow. An excellent beginning place for the parents of preemies and their families and friends. Internet only: http://www.comeunity.com/premature/

Preemie Resource Page: Large list of publications, organizations, Web sites, and other resources. Internet only: http://members.aol.com/MarAim/preemie.htm

After the NICU: Web site providing advice for parents of babies newly discharged from the NICU.
Internet only:
http://home.san.rr.com/gtbangs/advice.htm

The Alexis Foundation: a nonprofit foundation offering information and support services for parents of preemies, and involved in fund-raising to promote research into new treatments for premature in-fants. P.O. Box 1126, Birmingham, MI 48012-1126.
Phone: (877) ALEXIS-0. E-mail: thealexisfoundation@prodigy.net
World Wide Web:
http://pages.prodigy.net/thealexisfoundation/THEALEXIS1.html

American Association of Premature Infants (A.A.P.I.): a nonprofit, advocacy organization dedicated to improving the quality of health, developmental and educational services for premature infants, chil-dren and their families. P.O. Box 46371, Cincinnati, OH 45246-0371.
E-Mail: feedback@aapi-online.org
World Wide Web: http://www.aapi-online.org

Bissell's Homepage: offers information on two conditions often asso-ciated with premature birth: tracheotomies for home ventilation and cerebral palsy. Internet only: http://www.twinenterprises.com/bissell

Cerebral Palsy

National Institute of Neurological Disorders: provides information on the nature and treatment of cerebral palsy. P.O. Box 5801, Bethesda, MD 20824. Phone: (301) 496-5751 or (800) 352-9424. World Wide Web: http://www.ninds.nih.gov/patients/disorder/cp/cphtr.htm

Cerebral Palsy Multimedia Tutorial: Web site maintained by the Children's Medical Center of the University of Virginia gives a thorough introduction to the illness, its treatment and its impact on children. World Wide Web: http://hsc.virginia.edu/cmc/tutorials/cp/cp.htm

United Cerebral Palsy Association: Nation's second largest health-related charitable organization provides extensive information on cerebral palsy and other disabilities. 1660 L Street, NW, Suite 700, Washington, DC 20036. Phone: (800) USA-5UCP (872-5827). World Wide Web: http://www.ucpa.org

Retinopathy of Prematurity

ROP Support Group: Web site and e-mail discussion group on this serious eye disease related to premature birth, maintained by Dr. Scott Richards of the Country Hills Eye Center, 875 E. Country Hill, Ogden, UT 84403. Phone: (888) EYE-CNTR. World Wide Web: http://www.konnections.com/eyedoc/ropstart.html

Growing Strong: Internet site maintained by adult former preemie with ROP. Web site provides separate areas with descriptive information on ROP and support information for parents of visually impaired children. World Wide Web: http://www.growingstrong.org

Congenital Conditions

March of Dimes Birth Defects Foundation: Charitable organization provides extensive information, fact sheets and support services re-

lated to all genetic disorders. 1275 Mamaroneck Avenue, White Plains, NY 10605. Phone: (888) MODIMES.
E-mail: resourcecenter@modimes.org
World Wide Web: http://www.modimes.org

Genetic Alliance: Organization dedicated to providing information and support related to all genetic disorders. Internet site has a searchable database of support organizations broken down by literally every disorder that can affect a child. Information also available by mail or phone. 4301 Connecticut Avenue, NW, #404, Washington, DC 20008-2304. Phone: (800) 336-GENE.
E-mail: info@geneticalliance.org
World Wide Web: http://www.geneticalliance.org/

Association of Birth Defect Children: Charitable organization that provides phone information, written materials, special reports and newsletters to parents and professionals about all kinds of birth defects, resources, support groups and environmental exposures that may cause birth defects. Has extensive list of fact sheets and e-mail list. Internet only: http://www.birthdefects.org/

Cleft Palate Foundation: 104 South Estes Drive, Suite 204, Chapel Hill, NC 27514. Phone: (800) 242-5338. E-mail: clefline@aol.com
World Wide Web: http://www.cleft.com

Congenital Heart Anomalies-Support, Education and Resources, Inc.: 2112 North Wilkins Road, Swanton, OH 43558.
Phone: (419) 825-5575. E-mail: chaser@compuserve.com
World Wide Web: http://www.csun.edu/~hfmth006/chaser

American Heart Association: Extensive information on congenital heart diseases and treatments. 7272 Greenville Avenue, Dallas, Texas 75231. Phone: (800) AHA-USA1. World Wide Web:
http://www.americanheart.org/Heart_and_Stroke_A_Z_Guide/conghd.html

Cystic Fibrosis Foundation: 6931 Arlington Road, Second Floor, Bethesda, MD 20814. Phone: (800) 344-4823. E-mail: info@cff.org World Wide Web: http://www.cff.org

National Down Syndrome Society: Foundation provides extensive information and support for individuals with Down Syndrome, their parents and families. Comprehensive information on all aspects of the condition, related research, legislation and fact sheets. 666 Broadway, New York, NY 10012-2317. Phone: (800) 221-4602.
E-mail: info@ndss.org
World Wide Web: http://www.ndss.org

Myotonic & Congenital Dystrophy Support Group International: 185 Unionville Road, Freedom, PA 15042. E-Mail: tallships@usa.net World Wide Web:
http://www.angelfire.com/pa2/MyotonicDystrophy/index.html

Spina Bifida Association of America: 4590 MacArthur Boulevard., NW, Suite 250, Washington, DC 20007. Phone: (800) 944-3285.
E-mail: sbaa@sbaa.org
World Wide Web: http://www.sbaa.org

Support Organization for Trisomy 18, 13 and Related Disorders: 2982 South Union Street, Rochester, NY 14624. Phone: (800)716-SOFT. E-mail: barbsoft@aol.com
World Wide Web: http://www.trisomy.org

Other Conditions Seen in and after the NICU

National Information Center on Deafness: Gallaudet University, 800 Florida Avenue, NE, Washington, DC 20002.
Phone: (202) 651-5051. TDD: (202) 651-5052.
E-mail: nicd@gallua.gallaudet.edu

Gastrostomy Support: Information and support for parents of children with G-tubes and other digestive disorders. Internet only: http://www.challengenet.com/~g-tube/index2.spml

Hydrocephalus Association: 870 Market Street, Suite 705, San Francisco, CA 94102. Phone: (888) 598-3789. E-mail: hydroassoc@aol.com World Wide Web: http://www.hydroassoc.org

Intraventricular Hemorrhage (I.V.H. Parents): P.O. Box 56-1111, Miami, FL 33256. Phone: (305) 232-0381.
E-mail: ronlondner@worldnet.att.net

National Center for Learning Disabilities: 381 Park Avenue South, Suite 1401, New York, NY 10016. Phone: (888) 575-7373.
World Wide Web: http://www.ncld.org

The PVL Resource Center: Information on the neurological ailment, Periventricular Leukomalacia. 1195 Penfield Center Road, Penfield, NY 14526. E-mail: reenie@computer-connection.net World Wide Web: http://www.computer-connection.net/~reenie/index.htm

Miscellaneous

Neonatology on the Web: An Internet site geared to doctors but with copious information useful to parents of preemies and ill newborns as well, including a glossary of all neonatal medications.
Internet only:
http://www.neonatology.org/index.html

Center for the Study of Multiple Births: Suite 464, 333 East Superior Street, Chicago, IL 60611. Phone: (312) 908-9093.
E-mail: lgk395@nwu.edu
World Wide Web: http://www.multiplebirth.com/

Stages of Fetal Development, by Week:
Internet only:
http://www.babycenter.com/fetaldevelopment/

Miller Children's Hospital, Long Beach, CA: The setting for *Baby ER*.
World Wide Web: http://www.memorialcare.com/Miller/About.hfm

Index

Names preceded by * are pseudonyms.

About the Author

EDWARD HUMES, winner of the Pulitzer Prize and a PEN Center USA West award, is the author of five other books. He lives in Southern California.